PETER TATCHELL

AIDS
A GUIDE TO
SURVIVAL

PREFACE BY
DR CHARLES
FARTHING

To Chris
With Best Wishes
Peter Tatchell

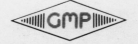

First published in July 1986 as a Heretic Book
    by GMP Publishers Ltd,
      PO Box 247, London N15 6RW
World copyright © 1986 Peter Tatchell
Preface world copyright © 1986 Charles Farthing

British Library Cataloguing in Publication Data

```
Tatchell, Peter
  AIDS: a guide to survival.
  1. AIDS (Disease)--Prevention--Handbooks,
  manuals, etc.
  I. Title
  614.5'993    RA644.A25
```

ISBN 0-946097-021-6

Illustrations by Louis Mackay
Photosetting by MC Typeset Ltd, 34 New Road, Chatham, Kent
Printed and bound by The Guernsey Press Ltd, Guernsey, C.I.

This book is dedicated to the memory of my former lover Peter Smith – jazz guitarist/saxophonist and socialist comrade – who was killed in an accident on 24 June 1985; and to all those brave people with AIDS who are fighting for their lives with determination and dignity – despite the hysteria, ignorance and prejudice of others around them, and despite the government's shameful record of neglect. Let their courage be an inspiration to us all.

Acknowledgements

In the course of preparing this book I have drawn on the published works and the assistance and advice of the following people and organisations to whom I am immensely grateful: Professor Michael Adler of the Middlesex Hospital for his helpful criticism of the draft manuscript; the AIDS Project of Los Angeles, especially Albert Ogle, Ted Tripella and John Mortimer and the editor, staff and contributors to *The Optimist*; Dr Erica Allason-Jones; the BBC 2 Open Space Programme *A Plague On You; Capital Gay* for its invaluable and unrivalled news documentation of the AIDS issue; Dr Charles Farthing of St Stephen's Hospital for his useful comments on the text; my editor at GMP David Fernbach; the Hall-Carpenter Gay and Lesbian Archives for access to their library facilities; Clyde Huff for his encouragement and regular supply of American source material; Dr Elizabeth Kubler-Ross, author of *On Death and Dying*; the Lesbian and Gay Media Project; Dr Arnold Linken; Joan Maddock; Penny Newell at the Southwark Welfare Rights Unit; Jo Ramsey of the Health Education Council; Justin Sibley; Dr Carl Simonton and Stephanie Simonton for their pioneering work in the field of psychosomatic health; Christopher Spence, author of the pamphlet *AIDS – An Issue for Everyone*; the staff and volunteers at the Terrence Higgins Trust; Mary Walker; David Watters at the Haemophilia Society; and to the following publications whose articles I have drawn upon: *American Scientist, British Medical Journal, The Lancet, Nature* and *New Scientist*.

Recommended further reading: *Getting Well Again* by Dr Carl Simonton; *The Will To Live* by Dr Arnold Hutschnecker; *Fighting For Our Lives* by Kit Mouat.

Special thanks to Kit Mouat, a founder member of the self-help group Cancer Contact, who has survived two bouts of cancer, the first of which was diagnosed way back in 1969! Despite her doctor's pessimistic prognosis, since then she has led a productive life, including the penning of poems of inspiration to people with life-threatening illnesses, such as the following:

On Being Told Bluntly That I Had 'Inoperable Secondary Cancers' in March 1982

Away with prognostic doom,
   there is no need for praying . . .
If that bloody surgeon says I'm going –
   I'm staying . . .

Contents

Preface by Dr Charles Farthing 7

Introduction 9
Chapter 1: Understanding AIDS 11
    What is AIDS? 11
    The Origin and Spread of AIDS 12
    The Cause of AIDS 14
    How AIDS Damages the Immune System 15
    AIDS-Induced Opportunistic Infections and Cancers 17
    The Symptoms of AIDS 19
    How Doctors Test for AIDS 20
    Methods of Transmitting AIDS 22
    Who is at Risk? 25
    Putting AIDS in Perspective 27
Chapter 2: Preventing AIDS 28
    Taking the HTLV-3 Test 28
    Protecting the Blood 30
    Safe Methods of Sex 31
Chapter 3: Fighting Back Against Aids 38
    Coping With Diagnosis 38
    The Will to Live 40
        A Positive Mental Attitude 41
        A Sense of Self-Esteem 43
        A Purpose or Goal in Life 44
        An Active Participation in Fighting Illness 45
    Mentally Fighting AIDS 47
        Meditation 49
        Mental Imagery 53
        Positive Mental Reinforcement 55
    Strengthening the Body's Physical Defences 60
        A Nutritious Vitamin-Fortified Diet 62
        Plenty of Exercise 70
        Regular Sleep 71
        Stress Reduction 73
    HTLV-3 and AIDS Support Groups 78
Chapter 4: Living With AIDS 80
    Self-Care and Home Hygiene 80
    Sustaining Sexual Relationships 83
    Home or Hospital? 84
    Patients' Rights 84
    Social Security Entitlements 85
    Facing the Possibility of Death 87
    Coping With Caring 91

Chapter 5: Campaigning to Defeat AIDS   95
    AIDS Discrimination   97
    Government Complacency   101
    Gay Responses   107
    A Programme of Action Against AIDS   111

Appendix 1: Day Planner   119
Appendix 2: Affirmation Meditation   120
Appendix 3: Relaxation Meditation   122
Appendix 4: Mental Imagery   124
Appendix 5: Work-Out   126
Appendix 6: Relaxation Exercises   132
Appendix 7: Qi Gong   135
Appendix 8: Body Massage   138
Appendix 9: Acupressure   141
Useful Contacts   143

Preface

AIDS is a new disease and a frightening one. Already it affects many thousands around the globe and many have died. The AIDS virus (HTLV III/LAV) is, however, far more widespread than the number of AIDS cases might suggest. Hundreds of thousands, perhaps several million people worldwide, currently carry HTLV III/LAV and an unknown percentage of them will develop the condition of AIDS over a course of anything from two to perhaps ten years or more. At the present time, the vast majority of these infected people are well or suffering only minor medical symptoms, but they face an uncertain future. A vaccine, if it can be developed, is unlikely to help those already infected and scientific hope rests on the discovery of an effective antiviral drug against the AIDS virus – HTLV III/LAV (or as recently renamed – "The Human Immunodeficiency Virus or HIV). With developments in molecular biology over recent years, there is good reason to be hopeful that such a drug will be found soon, but "soon" may easily be measured in years. Many patients want to know what they can do *now* to help themselves and Peter Tatchell addresses himself to this question. I am sure many sufferers of HTLV III/LAV infection will benefit considerably from reading his book.

There are many things a patient can do to improve his chances when affected by this virus. Perhaps the most important of all, however, is to have a positive attitude of mind and a will to live. All doctors know from caring for patients with other serious illnesses, such as cancer, that a patient with a strong desire to survive can often outlive all expectations, but conversely, a patient who gives up in despair may die with surprising suddenness. There are many ways that one may achieve a positive attitude of mind, and whatever path is taken it usually means taking a close look at one's life, defining one's goals, coming to terms with what is "the real self", and getting to like oneself. It also means getting adequate rest and not overstressing oneself at work or play. Many fears are definitely born of fatigue. We know for certain that depression and stress have a very deleterious effect on the immune system and alone can precipitate some of the very signs of immunodepression, such as shingles and eczema, that are seen in HTLV III/LAV disease. It is very important therefore that someone infected with this virus, whose immune system may already be impaired, does not further depress it by locking into despair or overwork.

There are many other things one can do to help oneself – eating a good diet, stopping such body-stressing activities as taking drugs like cocaine or amphetamines, making sure one gets a reasonable amount of exercise, and cutting down on exposure to other infections. It is possible that HTLV III/LAV is sometimes activated by episodes of other infections, especially venereal ones such as hepititis B and syphilis. Avoidance of such infections may necessitate a considerable change in lifestyle for some. Mr Tatchell gives all these things adequate coverage as well as discussing various alternative therapies. (For "alternative" medicine, though, I ask you to read "complementary medicine". Many patients may derive great benefit from their homeopathic doctor or acupuncturist but therapists in these other disciplines would agree that it is better they work with, rather than instead of, a conventional medical man.)

Finally, I would like to sound a note of caution. Already in the United Kingdom, two individuals have actually sent postal advertisements for certain cures for AIDS. Not surprisingly these have been expensive. Be cautious and evaluate carefully what you read. When it comes to any suggested drug therapy, even vitamin pills, discuss the tablets or medicines with your doctor first. Peter Tatchell by and large gives good advice – not everyone does.

Charles Farthing

Introduction

Untold spiritual strength and physical power lie within,
Sources of self-healing by nature begotten.
Chained and dormant for so long,
They lie inside us, forsaken and forgotten.
But as the Chariot of Death rides close and strong,
Now is the time to awaken those sleeping giants within.

This book is intended as a brief and simple guide to understanding, preventing and fighting back against AIDS. It is primarily aimed at people who are HTLV–3 antibody positive, or who have AIDS or the AIDS-related conditions of PGL and ARC. However, even people who are well will hopefully find its recommendations helpful for improving their health and enhancing the quality of their lives.

In contrast with the gloom and despair which is normally associated with AIDS, there is an alternative message of hope and optimism: AIDS is *not* inevitably fatal. People who are infected with the virus are *not* powerless and helpless. Instead of accepting their fate as passive victims who redefine themselves as 'patients' and slide irreversibly into the 'sick role', people with HTLV–3 infection and AIDS can make the conscious, positive choice to mentally and physically fight the disease. This method of resisting AIDS, which can usefully complement conventional medical treatment, is premised on the 'whole person' approach to health:

* The idea that illness is not a problem which is localised solely in a particular part of the body, and that it is not a purely physical thing; but that the mind, body and emotions are interrelated and interdependent parts of the person which interact to cause sickness and wellness.
* The view that instead of having a single simple cause, most illnesses involve a series of *negative* 'triggers' or 'co-factors' which combine to precipitate disease and impede the immune system's ability to destroy infection. Conversely, the restora-

9

tion of health also depends on the activation of multiple *positive* 'triggers' or 'co-factors'.

* The concept of the body as a self-regulating organism which can be induced to cure itself naturally of many diseases if the immune system is adequately stimulated so that it functions at full efficiency.
* The notion that the healing process should treat the person, not just the disease; and treat the deep, underlying roots of the illness rather than its superficial symptoms.

In the case of AIDS, for the full syndrome to develop, two things are necessary. First, the person must become infected with the HTLV–3 virus. Second, their immune system must be operating at under-efficiency and therefore be unable to repel the virus. Hence the rationale of fighting back against AIDS is to enhance immune functioning so that the body has a better chance of suppressing or destroying the HTLV–3 infection. This involves mentally fighting AIDS using the methods of meditation, mental imagery and positive mental reinforcement which indirectly improve immune efficiency. It also involves physically fighting AIDS by directly strengthening the body's immune system through switching to a 'healthy living' regime, including a nutritious vitamin-fortified diet, plenty of exercise, regular sleep and stress reduction via the practice of relaxation techniques. The aim is to thereby increase the sum total of mental and physical factors which favour maximum resistance to the AIDS virus, so that people with HTLV–3 infection can reduce their chances of developing full-blown AIDS, and those who already have AIDS can improve their prospects of survival and achieve happier and more satisfying lives. This is not a false hope or self-delusion. The fact that 90 percent of people infected with the HTLV–3 virus do not get AIDS is proof that the immune system *can* control and possibly even conquer the disease. Referring to the curative potential of each person's inner psychological and physiological resources, Dr Dick Richards asserts: 'We have an armoury of weapons to fight disease. We can use all or some . . . the more we use, the more chance we have of winning the battle.' That's what this approach to AIDS is all about – not simply relying on external medical treatment or any single panacea; but mobilising one's entire array of internal mental and bodily powers to wholeheartedly fight back against this disease with vigour and determination.

Chapter 1

Understanding AIDS

> With knowledge,
> understanding is gained,
> ignorance dispelled,
> prejudice confounded,
> and power unleashed.

What is AIDS?

AIDS stands for Acquired Immune Deficiency Syndrome. As its name suggests, AIDS is contracted rather than inherited; it results in immune inadequacy; and it consists of several associated symptoms and diseases.

Essentially, AIDS involves a weakening of the body's immune system so that its natural defence mechanisms are no longer able to fight off illness. The body then becomes vulnerable to specific types of life-threatening disease: viral, fungal, protozoal, and (occasionally) bacterial infections, as well as rare cancers. These are known as 'opportunistic' infections and cancers because they take advantage of the opportunity provided by the AIDS-damaged immune system to invade the body and rapidly multiply out of control – often with fatal consequences. Thus, strictly speaking, no one dies from AIDS. They are actually killed by opportunistic diseases which the AIDS-impaired body is unable to resist.

For the purposes of medical surveillance and diagnosis, AIDS is defined as follows. First, the presence of life-threatening opportunistic infections or cancers. Second, the simultaneous suppression of the body's immune system. And third, the absence of any other known illness such as leukemia which could cause and explain the immune deficiency. Additionally, though not yet part of the official definition, nearly everyone with AIDS shows evidence of infection by the virus known as HTLV-3 – Human T-cell Lymphotropic Virus type 3 – which has been identified as the cause of AIDS.

HTLV–3 is also the cause of two milder AIDS–linked illnesses which fall short of the full AIDS definition: Persistent Generalised Lymphadenopathy (PGL) and AIDS–Related Complex (ARC). HTLV–3 infection thus appears to result in a spectrum of three interconnected illnesses, ranging from PGL which is the least severe, to ARC which is fairly severe, and to AIDS which is the most severe. Though neither PGL nor ARC involve life–threatening opportunistic infections or cancers, they both include evidence of HTVL–3 infection and some of the symptoms of AIDS and can be precursors to the subsequent development of AIDS.

Comparatively speaking, PGL is quite mild. It entails prolonged swelling of the lymph glands in the groin, neck, shoulders and armpits for periods in excess of three months – sometimes with pain and sometimes without. On the other hand, ARC can be almost as debilitating as AIDS. It involves the presence of at least two of the symptoms typically associated with AIDS – substantial weight loss, extreme fatigue, persistent diarrhoea and fever, drenching night sweats and minor bouts of infections such as oral thrush and shingles. Although these ARC symptoms and infections are not life–endangering, they do indicate a significant degree of immune deficiency and can be a highly unpleasant experience. Whilst from 10 to 20 percent of people with PGL or ARC later go on to develop AIDS, some people develop AIDS without previously experiencing either PGL or ARC.

Contrary to popular mythology, AIDS does not always result in a swift and inevitable death. According to the American AIDS monitoring agency, the Centers for Disease Control, 15 percent of those diagnosed with AIDS in 1981 were still alive at the beginning of 1986.

The Origin and Spread of AIDS

From 1978 onwards, a strange unexplainable illness began appearing in the United States. At first, it was not realised that there was any connection between the separate cases and diverse symptoms. By June 1981, however, a tentative pattern began to emerge which led the Centers for Disease Control to officially propose the existence of a specific new illness. As evidence, the CDC pointed to 31 cases of rare skin cancers and pneumonic infections which were accompanied by unexplained immune abnormalities. Since nearly all the diagnosed individuals were homosexual or bisexual men, it was initially assumed that some aspect of gay people's lifestyle was to blame. Accordingly, the new disease was dubbed Gay-Related Immune Deficiency.

Soon afterwards, however, the disease was also discovered amongst heterosexual intravenous drug users who didn't fit the 'Gay-Related' pattern. This prompted the renaming of the disease as AIDS. Within a few months, this heterosexual trend was confirmed with the diagnosis of AIDS amongst Haitian immigrants and haemophiliac recipients of blood transfusions.

Since then, it has become apparent that AIDS is not a sudden new illness. Judging from retrospective analysis of medical reports and blood samples taken in the early 1970s, it seems that AIDS has been prevalent, but unrecognised, in several Central African countries for at least the last fifteen years.

Currently, the existence of AIDS and HTLV–3 infection is positively confirmed on a substantial scale in Zaire, Central African Republic, Zambia, Rwanda, Burundi, Uganda, Kenya and Tanzania. Contrary to the view that AIDS is a 'gay disease', in these countries AIDS is almost entirely heterosexually transmitted. In addition to mainly affecting heterosexuals, it also affects women as much as men, and children as well as adults.

The connection of AIDS with Africa has been further strengthened by the discovery that a virus similar to HTLV–3 appears to be routinely present in the Green Monkey population of central Africa. This has given rise to the following informed, but as yet *unproven*, theory about the origins of AIDS:

About twenty years ago, it is suggested, an AIDS-type virus which exists harmlessly amongst Green Monkeys crossed over into the human population in the rural areas of equatorial Africa where it mutated into the HTLV–3 virus. Assisted by the process of rural migration to urban areas and the more liberal sexual morality in large African cities like Kinshasa, the virus spread via heterosexual contact and from mother to foetus in the womb.

From Africa, the HTLV–3 virus was spread to the United States via Haiti. During the 1970s, many Haitians who had been migrant workers in central Africa returned to Haiti infected with HTLV–3. There being a significant incidence of bisexuality amongst Haitians, they then passed the virus into the US gay community through homosexual contact with American gay and bisexual men. This contact occurred both via US tourists holidaying in Haiti, and also via Haitian immigration into the United States.

Once established in the American gay community, with its more frequent change of sexual partners and slightly more vulnerable sexual practices, the virus multiplied and dispersed more rapidly than ever before. From the USA, the virus spread to Europe, partly through the importation of tainted American blood products, but primarily as a result of sexual contact between American and European gay men – except in France and Belgium where heterosexual contact with central African partners has been a major channel of infection.

In Britain, the first case of AIDS was diagnosed in December 1981 and the first death occurred in July 1982. By the spring of 1986, there had been 380 cases of AIDS and nearly 200 deaths. Estimates of the number of British people infected with the HTLV–3 virus vary from 20,000 to 50,000. Worldwide, the number of cases of AIDS reported in mid-1986 was 30,000. However, the true figure is probably much higher as some East European and Third World countries refuse to admit they have any cases of AIDS.

The Cause of AIDS

AIDS is caused by a virus called Human T-cell Lymphotropic Virus type 3. For brevity, it is simply referred to as HTLV–3 or the AIDS virus. It gets its name because it damages the immune system by infecting a particular group of lymphocytes in the bloodstream – the T helper cells. The HTLV–3 virus has to get inside this particular group of cells in order to multiply and undermine the immune system.

HTLV–3 was first discovered in 1983. It is the third in a series of recently detected human retroviruses. Of the other two, HTLV–1 is linked with human T-cell leukemia and HTLV–2 has been isolated from a case of hairy cell leukemia. Other retroviruses occur amongst animals and cause similar immune deficiencies to HTLV–3. This happens in the case of cats infected by Feline Leukemia Virus and Macaque monkeys infected by Simian T-Lymphotropic Virus type 3.

HTLV–3 does its damage by fundamentally disrupting the genetic structure of the cells it attacks. Being a retrovirus, once it has invaded a T helper cell, HTLV–3 'reverse transcribes' its genetic code into the T helper cell's DNA. This induces the T helper cell to make the components which enable new HTLV–3 viruses to form and then disperse throughout the bloodstream to invade and infect other T helper cells. In effect, HTLV–3 transforms the T helper cells into mini virus factories. Instead of reproducing themselves, the T helper cells reproduce HTLV–3 viruses and this causes the progressive decline of the body's T helper cell population. As more and more T helper cells are destroyed, the immune system steadily collapses.

The average incubation time between initial infection with the HTLV–3 virus and the onset of AIDS is 3–4 years, though it can vary from as little as 6 months to as long as 6 years. Not everyone infected with the virus develops AIDS. Most infected people stay healthy. Only about 25 per cent later fall ill – 10 per cent with AIDS and 15 per cent with Persistent Generalised Lymphadenopathy or AIDS-Related Complex.

Though HTLV–3 is the cause of AIDS, and though infection results in the production of HTLV-3 antibodies, not everyone with AIDS shows HTLV–3 antibodies in their blood when tested. This is because the antibodies decline and become difficult to detect in certain circumstances, especially when the severity of AIDS increases in its advanced stages of development.

How AIDS Damages the Immune System

The immune system is the body's natural defence against disease. Its cells seek out, identify and destroy viruses and other foreign invaders which enter the body, as well as infected cells and the body's own abnormal or malignant cells which can cause cancers.

This role is primarily carried out by a particular class of white blood cells, the lymphocytes. There are two main types of lymphocyte cells in the bloodstream – B cells and T cells. They each have different functions and capabilities and this gives rise to two different but interrelated systems of immune defence.

T cell immune defence

The T cells are the main command and control centre of the immune system. There are three kinds of T cells – T helper cells, T suppressor cells and T killer cells.

The T cell immune defence begins with a special type of scavenger cell, the macrophages. They identify the foreign invaders and then inform the T helper cells. The T helper cells respond by switching on the immune system – activating B cells to produce antibodies and T killer cells to destroy the foreign invaders and, if necessary, any of the body's cells which have become infected or malignant.

Once the foreign invaders have been defeated, the T suppressor cells switch off the immune system, thereby deactivating the T helper, T killer and B cells.

B cell immune defence

In some cases, the B cells' defences are self-activating. In other cases they need to be stimulated into action by T helper cells. When an activated B cell encounters a foreign invader, it clones itself to create enlarged plasma cells. These plasma cells produce and secrete millions of antibodies. Some antibodies can directly destroy foreign invaders, whilst others act indirectly by coating the invaders and thereby making them palatable for scavenger cells to engulf and destroy.

Other cell immune defence

There are four other types of defender cells which act as support arms to the T and B cell immune defences. Natural killer cells get their name because they kill foreign invaders and infected and malignant cells spontaneously without any prior stimulation by the T helper cells. Macrophages, monocytes and granulo-

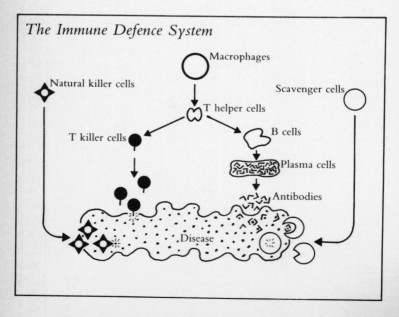

The Immune Defence System

cytes are three different varieties of scavenger cell which digest and destroy foreign invaders.

The effect of AIDS

The HTLV–3 virus is able to avoid destruction by the immune system and do the body's immunity lasting damage. It does this by entering the bloodstream where it infects and dramatically reduces the number of T helper cells – the lynchpins of the whole immune defence system. Instead of T helper cells outnumbering T suppressor cells by two to one as is normal in a healthy person, with AIDS the ratio is reversed. Since the T suppressor cells are unaffected by the virus, their volume remains at its normal level. In contrast, however, the population of T helper cells can be so seriously depleted that they are difficult to detect. Thus, the AIDS virus fundamentally alters the balance between the T helper cells which activate the immune system and the T suppressor cells which deactivate it.

In such circumstances, the depleted and weakened T helper cells are unable to properly switch on the immune system to resist the HTLV–3 virus or the opportunistic infections and cancers which follow. As a result, without adequate T helper cell stimulation, the T killer cells cannot destroy the foreign invaders, some of the B cells cannot produce the right antibodies in sufficient quantities, and even the response of the scavenger and natural killer cells is somewhat inhibited.

Although the T helper cells are the primary target of the AIDS virus, it appears that eventually the B cells and macrophages can also become infected. Once the virus enters the bloodstream and infects these various cells, it is transported by the blood to all parts of the body – skin tissues, organs, faeces and other body fluids.

There is some evidence that the T helper cells are most vulnerable to HTLV–3 infection when they are already multiplying in reaction to another serious infection such as hepatitis B. This seems to suggest that people whose immune systems are already damaged or under stress are more susceptible to AIDS.

AIDS-Induced Opportunistic Infections and Cancers

When the body's immune system is seriously impaired by AIDS, it is no longer able to effectively resist and repel illness. As a result, a whole series of diseases which would ordinarily be easily overcome by a healthy person instead spread unchecked and become life-threatening.

There are two types of disease which occur in people with AIDS – cancers which cause a minority of AIDS deaths, and opportunistic infections which account for the overwhelming majority of AIDS fatalities.

Of the cancers, the most prevalent is the normally rare skin tumour, Kaposi's Sarcoma. It is, in fact, not a new form of cancer, having been known to exist for more than a century. In its classical form, Kaposi's Sarcoma is usually slow-growing, non-fatal, and normally only affects elderly men of Jewish and Mediterranean descent. For the last sixty years, another form of Kaposi's Sarcoma has also been observed in central Africa where it affects young people of both sexes and sometimes results in death. The more recently discovered AIDS-related form of Kaposi's Sarcoma is the most aggressive. In addition to external skin lesions, it can also appear on the internal mucous membranes. Occasionally, it spreads to the lymph nodes, lungs and other bodily organs.

Primary lymphoma of the brain is another comparatively unusual cancer. It involves internal cerebral swelling and tumours which can precipitate convulsions, paralysis, partial blindness and personality disorders, including loss of memory and intelligence.

The other category of AIDS-induced diseases – the opportunistic infections – can be caused by four varieties of organism:

Protozoa. Pneumocystis Carinii Pneumonia (PCP) is a severe chest infection and the most common of all the opportunistic diseases. Toxoplasmosis Gondii causes inflammation and abscesses on the brain. Cryptosporidium Enteritis, Giardia Lablia and Entamoeba Histolytica are intestinal parasites which result in chronic diarrhoea and the malabsorption of food.

Viruses. Herpes Simplex I and II cause cold sores and genital herpes. Herpes Zoster – otherwise known as shingles – consists of painful skin eruptions and is due to the reactivation of a chickenpox virus which has laid dormant in the body since childhood. Epstein-Barr Virus results in glandular fever. Cytomegalovirus – which is usually referred to as CMV and is the most common opportunistic infection after PCP – can cause pneumonia, blindness and severe diarrhoea.

Fungi. Candida Albicans – or thrush as it is commonly known – is a yeast infection which affects the mouth, gastro-intestinal tract and occasionally the internal organs. Cryptococcus Neoformans invades the lungs to cause pneumonia and spreads to the brain where it results in meningitis.

Bacteria. Mycobacterium Avium Intracellularae is a tuberculosis-like illness which infects the bloodstream, lymph nodes, bone marrow, gut and other internal organs. Salmonella and Shigella Flexneri cause intestinal infections and diarrhoea. By comparison to protozoal, viral and fungal infections, these bacterial diseases are relatively rare amongst people with AIDS.

Of all these cancers and opportunistic infections, two diseases – Kaposi's Sarcoma and Pneumocystis Carinii Pneumonia – account for 70 percent of all AIDS diagnoses. Few people with PCP survive for more than two years, whilst 60 percent of those with Kaposi's Sarcoma alone survive for three years after diagnosis.

The Symptoms of AIDS

The development of AIDS-induced opportunistic infections and the AIDS-linked illnesses PGL and ARC variously involve at least one of the following symptoms:

* Indefinitely swollen glands in the neck, shoulders, armpits or groin.
* Profound and long-lasting fatigue.
* Unexplained weight loss of more than 5 kilos within two months.
* Prolonged loss of appetite.
* Persistent fevers or drenching night sweats.
* Long-term shortness of breath and dry cough.
* Frequent diarrhoea or bloody faeces.
* Thick white spots or coating over the tongue, gums or throat – normally accompanied by soreness and difficulty in swallowing.
* Unusual skin rashes or discolourations or cold sores.
* Severe headaches or nausea or dizziness.

Additionally, the two AIDS-related cancers result in the following distinct and defined symptoms:

* Kaposi's Sarcoma consists of new pink, purple or brown discolourations on or just under the skin – or sometimes in the mouth, nasal passages, intestines, rectum, or under the eyelids. These can either be flat like bruises, or raised in the form of lumps, nodules or blister-like swellings. They are normally painless and may grow larger and spread to other parts of the body.

* Lymphomas of the brain result in continuous or repeated bouts of blurred vision, severe headaches, mental disorientation, fits and personality changes.

People with one or more of these symptoms should not be alarmed, but seek a medical opinion to determine whether they are due to a common and minor illness, or to something more serious.

It is advisable to go direct to the Sexually Transmitted Diseases (STD) clinic at a local hospital rather than to a neighbourhood GP. STD doctors are more experienced and proficient in the diagnosis of AIDS. If required, they have access to the latest available treatments which they prescribe and administer free of charge. And at an STD clinic, patients' medical records are subject to stricter confidentiality.

How Doctors Test for AIDS

The presence of AIDS is not easy to diagnose. There is no single definitive test. Instead, it is necessary to undertake a series of procedures which check for evidence of the HTLV–3 virus and antibodies, as well as opportunistic infections, cancers and immune deficiency.

Test for the HTLV–3 virus

Though technically difficult and not widely available, it is now possible using blood samples to directly look for and identify the HTLV–3 virus which causes AIDS.

Test for HTLV–3 antibodies

When the HTLV–3 virus invades the body, the immune system produces specific antibodies to attack it. These antibodies persist indefinitely in the blood. The HTLV–3 antibody test shows whether or not any antibodies to the virus are present. If they are – a positive result – it is evidence that the person concerned has at some point been infected by the HTLV–3 virus and is probably still infectious. If no antibodies are detected – a negative result – this usually means that the person has not been infected. However, there is a delay between the date of infection and the production of significant quantities of antibodies. Normally, this delay is from four to eight weeks, though in some cases it can be as long as nine months. During this period, a person could be infected with the virus, but show no evidence of antibodies and register a negative result. Additionally, in some advanced cases of AIDS, HTLV–3 antibodies decline and become difficult to detect. In such circumstances, people can also record a negative test result.

Tests for opportunistic cancers and infections

* A biopsy consists of removing a small sample of skin or internal organ and is used to verify the existence of diseases such as Kaposi's Sarcoma and Pneumocystis Carinii Pneumonia (PCP).
* A viral culture involves incubating samples of blood, semen or urine which can then be microscopically examined to check for viruses like Cytomegalovirus (CMV).
* A faecal examination is used to determine the presence of Giardia Lablia and other intestinal infections.
* A blood sample is taken to look directly for the presence of infective agents such as Cryptococcus Neoformans, or indirectly for their antibodies as in the case of Epstein–Barr Virus.
* A chest X–ray is performed to detect signs of lung infections, especially PCP.
* An endoscopy is the insertion of a small flexible tube into the upper or lower end of the gastro–intestinal tract, or bronchial tubes, to search for signs of internal Kaposi's Sarcoma and infections such as thrush.
* A lumbar puncture drains samples of cerebral fluid from the spinal column to analyse for the presence of central nervous system infections such as Toxoplasmosis and Cryptococcus.
* An aspiration sucks out samples of sputum from deep inside the windpipe or lungs which can then be scrutinised for traces of CMV or PCP infection.

Tests for immune deficiency

* A total white blood cell count checks the number of white cells in the blood. In a fully operational immune system, it is usually in the range of 3,500–10,000 cells per millilitre of blood. Fewer than 3,500 white blood cells can indicate a possible susceptibility to, and presence of, opportunistic infections.
* A total lymphocyte count is similar. The lymphocytes are a

particular subset of white blood cells mainly made up of T and B cells. A combined total of more than 1,500 lymphocytes is normal for a healthy person. When the number is lower than 1,000 it is a sign of immune malfunctioning and vulnerability to disease. Everyone with opportunistic infections, and half those with Kaposi's Sarcoma, have a total lymphocyte count of less than 1,000.

* A quantitative immunoglobulin test measures the levels of all five classes of antibodies in the blood. Since the levels are frequently raised in people with AIDS, the presence of more of these antibodies than normal points to the possibility of infection by the HTLV–3 virus.

* A T-cell subset test analyses the number and ratio of T helper cells to T suppressor cells. Ordinarily, there are twice as many T helpers as there are T suppressors. With AIDS, however, the T helper cell population is drastically depleted and this results in T suppressors being in the majority. In this particular test, the probable existence of AIDS is indicated by a level of T helper cells which is lower than and substantially outnumbered by T suppressor cells.

* A delayed hypersensitivity skin test involves the injection of a small amount of a harmless, inactivated virus or bacteria into the skin of the forearm to determine the body's reaction. An absence of reaction indicates a degree of immune dysfunction and is frequently found in people with opportunistic infections and Kaposi's Sarcoma.

Methods of Transmitting AIDS

The AIDS virus, HTLV–3, damages the immune system by attacking a particular group of cells in the bloodstream – the T helper cells. To do this, it first has to get into the blood via a break in the skin or the internal mucous membranes of the eyes, nose, mouth, gastro-intestinal tract, urethra, vagina or rectum. Without a break caused by a cut, scratch, needle puncture, split, ulcer or open sore, the virus cannot get into the blood.

Once, however, the virus succeeds in entering the bloodstream it rapidly multiplies. Subsequently, it can be dispersed by the blood to all parts of the body, including the skin tissues, organs, faeces and other body fluids such as tears, saliva, urine, vaginal secretions and *especially semen* – though outside of semen and blood, the virus is found in much less concentrated quantities. Since the sole capacity of HTLV–3 is to destroy T helper cells in the bloodstream, the other diverse bodily regions and fluids are not harmed by its presence. They can, however, become infectious to varying degrees and capable of transmitting the virus to other people if, and only if, they come into *direct contact* with a break in the skin or internal mucous membranes.

This effectively rules out the transmission of AIDS by any form of everyday social contact such as shaking hands, using the same telephone or launderette, sharing toilet or canteen facilities, or even being in close proximity to the cough or sneeze of a person with AIDS. Although a sneeze, for example, could contain infectious nasal fluid, the virus would be present in very minute quantities and it would have to fall directly on an open wound or sore to have any chance of entering the blood and causing infection. The probability of this happening is virtually nil. Indeed, there has never been a single recorded case of AIDS being transmitted by sneezing or any other form of everyday social contact. Even more convincing: of all the doctors and health-care workers who regularly deal with AIDS patients, none have ever been infected in the course of their work by routine contact such as medical interviews, physical examinations, or the sharing of hospital facilities. The small number of medical staff who have contracted the virus have done so by accidentally pricking themselves with infected needles. If HTLV–3 was highly contagious, a large number of doctors and nurses in contact with AIDS patients would have now been infected. That fact that this has not happened is proof that the virus is not very infectious.

The methods, therefore, by which the virus is spread are primarily intimate sexual contact and the exchange of blood.

Sexual transmission

Sexual contact – both homosexual and heterosexual – is the most frequent method of transmitting AIDS. It accounts for 70 percent of American cases and 90 percent of cases in Britain.

Of the different types of sexual activity, vaginal and anal intercourse is overwhelmingly the most common mode of transmission, with the penetrated partner being at greatest risk of infection. This is because semen is a much more concentrated and mobile transporter of the virus than the relatively small quantities of blood and other fluids which are present in the vagina and rectum; and because the vaginal and rectal mucous membranes are slightly weaker and more prone to tissue breakage than the stronger skin which covers the penis. Thus, although the reverse process of transmission – from penetrated to penetrative partner – can occur, it is more difficult. It requires a break in the skin of the penis to be directly exposed to infected blood, or other infected fluid, in the vagina or the rectum.

Comparing the two forms of sexual intercourse, the AIDS virus is probably a little more readily transmitted via anal sex. Though minor tissue damage – usually so small that it's difficult to detect – routinely occurs during both homosexual and heterosexual intercourse, the rectal membrane tends to be slightly less strong and therefore quite often subject to minute tears and splits. Additionally, it consists of masses of tiny surface blood vessels which can be burst by the pressure and friction of the sex act, and occasionally by the strain of bowel movements which can directly contaminate faeces with blood. In contrast, though the vagina is also liable to tissue breakage, it is a bit stronger than the rectal membrane and this makes it marginally more difficult for the virus to be contracted heterosexually.

Some doctors, however, now dissent from this view. They argue that there is no qualitative difference between the composition of the vaginal and rectal membranes, and that both are sufficiently porous to permit the transmission of the HTLV–3 virus without requiring any breakage in the membrane surface to occur.

Most other types of sexual activity which involve an exchange of body fluids, such as kising and oral sex, can also transmit AIDS: though probably less easily than vaginal and anal intercourse because the virus is much less concentrated in saliva and oral contact involves less likelihood of mucous membrane damage. The danger in kissing and oral sex is that the virus could be passed on by infected semen and saliva entering the bloodstream via scratches or sores on the lips, gums, tongue or throat. If, however, it is swallowed into the gastro–intestinal tract, the virus is probably destroyed by the stomach's powerful acids. In oral sex, reverse infection could take place if the penis was subjected to teeth grazes and infected saliva then got into the abrasion. The only route of infectivity in mutual masturbation is if AIDS-contaminated semen falls directly on an open skin wound.

Blood transmission

Needle punctures. At present the most common method of direct blood transmission of AIDS is through the sharing of needles and syringes by people who inject drugs into their veins.

The virus can also be passed on via the use of infected acupuncture, ear-piercing or tattooing needles.

Transfusions. In the past, blood-borne AIDS was largely passed on from one person to another through the transfusion of infected whole blood, or plasma and blood products such as Factor 8 and Factor 9 which are used by haemophiliacs to remedy genetic deficiencies in their blood. Nowadays, by testing all donated blood and heat-treating plasma and Factors 8 and 9, the contamination of the blood supply has been almost entirely eliminated. The only possible remaining route of AIDS infection via blood transfusion is in the very unlikely case of an unwitting virus carrier donating blood in the period immediately after infection, but before the production of antibodies – in which case an HTLV–3 antibody test would show a negative result and the contaminated blood would therefore be certified fit for use in transfusions.

Other transmission

Mother to foetus. An infected mother can transmit the virus to her foetus in the womb or infect her new-born child through HTLV–3 contaminated breast milk.

Transplants. The transplant of infected tissue and organs has in the past transferred the virus to the recipient. However, today this is most unlikely as transplant donors are now screened for HTLV–3 infection.

Artificial insemination. Likewise with artificial insemination. Though mothers and foetuses have previously been infected by this method, the introduction of tests for all semen donors will eliminate it in the future.

Who Is At Risk?

The people who are at risk of contracting AIDS are those who do things which are known to cause the transmission of the virus, plus the sexual partners of such people. Essentially, this means that those at risk of AIDS infection are people who exchange body fluids – especially blood and semen.

Gay and bisexual men, particularly those who have anal sex, are the biggest risk group in the population. They comprise 65 percent of all people with AIDS in the USA and 85 percent of AIDS patients in Britain. By 1986, more than a third of gay men tested at London STD clinics were shown to be infected with the

HTLV–3 virus. By contrast, in Africa AIDS is overwhelmingly passed on heterosexually, both from men to women and from women to men. This global variability in the prevalence of heterosexually and homosexually transmitted AIDS is solely due to the fact that the virus originated in Africa amongst heterosexuals, but when it spread to the West, gay men were the first group within the population to be infected. Their frequency and types of sexual practice have made gay men more vulnerable to infection and resulted in the virus spreading more rapidly amongst homosexuals than heterosexuals. In the last couple of years, however, the number of heterosexual AIDS cases in the West has been steadily rising.

Haemophiliacs are the second largest risk group in Britain, with nearly 44 percent of people with Type A haemophilia currently registering a positive result to the HTLV–3 antibody test. However, the heat treatment of Factors 8 and 9 should now prevent the occurrence of any further cases of infection via blood products amongst haemophiliacs.

Blood transfusion recipients and people who received plasma prior to the introduction of blood donor screening in October 1985 run a small risk of contracting AIDS. There is a slightly higher risk of infection for those who received transfusions between 1979 when the virus first began to spread within Britain and 1984 when the government first called on AIDS risk groups not to donate blood. Blood donor testing for HTLV–3 should in future eliminate the spread of AIDS through transfusions.

Central African heterosexuals are another substantial group at risk. In some equatorial African countries, between 2 and 12 percent of the general population have been exposed to the AIDS virus and now carry antibodies. Amongst prostitute women – the highest African risk category – the rate of antibody positives is between 50 and 88 percent.

Drug users who share needles are proportionately the most rapidly growing risk group in Britain. In some major cities, nearly 50 percent of intravenous drug users now test HTLV–3 positive, and in Edinburgh the figure is 60 percent.

Prostitute women are still a relatively small risk group in Britain. So far, they have mainly been affected by AIDS not through sexual transmission, but because many prostitutes are also intravenous drug users.

Children born to infected parents are another fairly small risk group; though as the number of people infected with the virus grows, so will the number of babies born with congenital HTLV–3 infection.

Sexual partners of risk groups are a risk group in themselves and potentially the largest risk group of all. They include anyone who, in the last seven years, has had sexual relations with gay or bisexual men, haemophiliacs, blood transfusion recipients, heterosexuals from Central Africa, intravenous drug users or prostitute women.

Putting AIDS in Perspective

AIDS certainly is a serious and debilitating illness. Indeed, it is often fatal. But it is also a rare disease which is difficult to catch. Unlike a cold or measles, it is not highly contagious. It can only be transmitted in certain special circumstances: through intimate contact with a person carrying the virus and the virus entering the bloodstream via a break in the skin or internal mucous membranes.

For the general population, the risk of getting AIDS is extremely small. By spring 1986, out of a population of 56 million people there had been less than 400 cases of AIDS and less than 200 deaths. Compare this with the statistics for other causes of death in Britain during 1985: 190,000 from heart disease, 134,000 from cancer, 86,500 from respiratory infection, 5,000 from road accidents and 4,500 from diabetes. Thus, the average person has a much higher chance of killing themselves through tobacco smoking, careless driving, excessive alcohol consumption or a high-fat and high-sugar diet.

For people in the AIDS risk groups, however, the probability of contracting the virus is much higher, as the following two examples illustrate. Amongst intravenous drug users in Edinburgh, the rate of HTLV–3 infection is 60 percent. Thus, within this group a person who shares needles stands well over a 1 in 2 chance of infection. Since more than a third of gay men tested at London STD clinics are HTLV–3 antibody positive, on average every third sexual encounter with a person from this group will run the risk of infection unless both partners practise safe sex.

Chapter 2
Preventing AIDS

An ounce
of prevention
is worth
a pound of cure
and a ton
of regret.

Taking the HTLV–3 Test

Since October 1985, hospital STD clinics have made the
HTLV–3 antibody test generally available to people from AIDS
risk groups such as gay and bisexual men, haemophiliacs and
intravenous drug users, plus their sexual partners. The test
determines whether or not antibodies to the AIDS virus are
present. A positive result indicates the existence of antibodies
and shows that the person concerned has been infected with the
virus at some point in the past and that they are probably still
infectious.

The current antibody test is fairly reliable. Its failure rate is
only 1 out of every 300 tests performed. A false positive result,
which wrongly indicates the presence of antibodies, is usually
uncovered and corrected by the practice of double-checking
positive results, and wherever there is a doubt, repeating the test
using another method. If there are personal case histories or
symptoms which alert doctors to the possibility of infection, a
false negative result, which mistakenly records the absence of
antibodies, can be discovered and rectified by testing directly for
the virus itself.

The HTLV–3 antibody test does, however, have a number of
limitations. A positive result, for example, leaves open whether
the virus is still present, or whether it has been destroyed. Nor
does it show whether the person concerned will be one of the 10
percent of infected people who later go on to develop AIDS.

The test also has some drawbacks in that a positive result can sometimes provoke extreme anxiety and depression and be misused as an instrument of discrimination. Currently, for example, some people who are antibody positive are being refused life insurance, mortgages and hospital treatment; whilst others have been sacked from their jobs, evicted from flats or ostracised by their family, friends and fellow employees. On the other hand, there are some circumstances in which taking the test can be advantageous and advisable. Already it is mandatory for blood, sperm and organ donors. It would also be a sensible precaution for people at risk who are contemplating a family, given that the immune suppression involved in pregnancy increases the likelihood of an infected mother developing AIDS, and that infected parents can pass the virus from one generation to the next during conception, pregnancy and breast feeding.

People who are intensely worried about the possibility of infection are another group who may benefit from taking the test and clarifying their antibody status. For these people, knowing the truth one way or another may be preferable to the anxiety, and even ill health, which the uncertainty of not knowing can sometimes provoke. Testing could also be worthwhile in the case of a relationship where one partner is antibody positive and the other partner's status is unknown. In this situation, testing can contribute to an informed decision about sexual practices. In the event of a test revealing one partner to be negative, a switch to safe methods of sex could help ensure that he or she remains that way.

Beyond these specific categories of people, there are good reasons why others at risk ought also to consider taking the HTLV–3 antibody test. Ultimately, ignorance is never a good thing, and often it's simply an expression of self-denial. Since knowledge is power, taking the test and knowing the result enables informed decisions to be made which enhance a person's sense of control and mastery over their future. Thus, having a full awareness of one's antibody status not only often leads to wiser decisions and behaviour, but also to greater self-confidence. Certainly, most people who have taken the test report no regrets. For many, it has helped 'concentrate the mind', encouraging them to face the issue of AIDS head-on for the first time and acting as a catalyst for their adoption of less risky sexual practices: those who test positive tend to switch to safe sex out of a desire not to pass the virus on to others, whilst those who test negative tend to switch to safe sex out of a desire to stay that way.

But perhaps the most important advantage of taking the test is that if a person knows they are infected with the virus, there are constructive things they can do to reduce their chances of developing full-blown AIDS. These include building up their physical and psychological strength through meditation, mental imagery, and a healthy living regime of nutritious diet, regular sleep and exercise, stress limitation, and drug and alcohol reduction. Of course, everyone *ought* to live healthily anyway. However, it is often the case that people are more likely to make these constructive changes in their lifestyle if they know they are antibody positive and have to face up to the possibility of a life-threatening illness.

Protecting the Blood

The direct exchange of blood from one person to another is the surest and quickest route of transmitting the HTLV–3 virus. For this reason, to protect the blood transfusion service and its recipients the following groups of people at risk from AIDS are advised not to donate blood or plasma:

* Gay and bisexual men, or any man who has had a homosexual experience since 1979.
* Haemophiliacs in receipt of Factors 8 and 9.
* Blood or plasma transfusion recipients over the six years prior to October 1985 when donor testing began.
* Central African heterosexuals.
* Intravenous drug users, plus any former users who have injected themselves since 1979.
* Prostitute women, including women who have been prostitutes at any time since 1979.
* The sexual partners of the above risk groups, again dating back to 1979.

There is virtually no danger of blood-borne AIDS transmission through medical or dental treatment, as all equipment is either sterilised or disposable and all blood donations are now tested for HTLV–3 infection. However, there is a possible risk of infection from High Street ear-piercers, tattooists and some acupuncturists – not all of whom maintain adequate standards of hygiene and needle sterilisation.

So far as intravenous drug users are concerned, a major reason for the spread of AIDS amongst this section of the population has in fact been the government's crackdown on drugs. This has included a policy of drastically restricting the over-the-counter availability of syringes and needles in chemists shops. This policy has not, however, stopped people injecting drugs. Instead, it has prompted a brisk black market trade in secondhand injection equipment and resulted in the increased sharing of needles. Shooting up drugs and swapping needles is always hazardous. The only sure way to be safe is not to inject drugs at all. However, those who continue to use intravenous drugs can reduce their risk of infection from AIDS and other diseases by taking the following precautions. First, acquire your own syringe and needle set and don't share it with anyone else. Second, wash and disinfect the skin before injecting. And third, clean the injection set with surgical spirit after each use and then keep it in a clean sealed container until it is next required.

Safe Methods of Sex

Nowadays, all blood donations are screened for the HTLV–3 virus. So outside the relatively small number of people who inject drugs, hardly any new cases of direct blood-borne AIDS transmission are likely to occur in years to come. Overwhelmingly, future HTLV-3 infection will be sexually transmitted.

In the absence of a vaccine or cure for AIDS, prevention is the only certain way by which people at risk and their sexual partners can safeguard their health. Prevention does not, however, require celibacy. The choice is not between AIDS or abstinence. It is between AIDS and playing safely. Safe sex involves having sex in ways which cannot transmit the virus and avoiding forms of sex which can pass on infection. Essentially, this means sticking to sexual activities which don't allow blood, semen, saliva or faeces to get into another person's body. The key to playing safe and preventing AIDS is not how often people have sex or how many sexual partners they have. It is the *way* people have sex. If people play dangerously, they can contract AIDS from a one-off sexual experience. On the other hand, if people play safely, they can have as much sex with as many different partners as they want, yet not be at risk of infection.

The relative safety or danger of various sexual activities is as follows:

Playing dangerously

* Oral, anal or vaginal sex without a condom.
* Sucking or tonguing the anus or vagina.

* Sharing douches, enemas or sex toys such as vibrators.
* Fist fucking.
* Sadomasochism which draws blood.
* Urination or water sports which enter the body.

Playing riskily

* Mouth-to-mouth French kissing.
* Thigh or buttock fucking.
* Fingering a partner's anus or vagina.

Playing safely

* Caressing, hugging and cuddling.
* Massage.
* Body kissing.
* Mutual or group masturbation.
* Body-to-body rubbing.
* Oral, anal or vaginal sex using a condom.
* Self-fingering of the anus or vagina.
* Sadomasochism without breaking the skin.

Playing safely begins with *checking the body and covering any breaks in the skin*. Cuts, sores, cracks or grazes should be protected with a waterproof plaster so that semen from mutual masturbation, or saliva from body kissing, is unable to penetrate into the bloodstream.

Nail manicuring is a sensible precaution since long or damaged nails can cause minor scratches and cuts, especially during the fingering of the anus or vagina.

Douching before showering and sex can slightly reduce the chances of picking up infected matter during internal finger lubrication and stimulation. In the case of anal sex, douching can also remove residual hardened faeces which might damage a condom. It is advisable, however, not to share douches with a partner and to only use those with smooth rounded nozzles so as to protect the body's delicate mucous membranes from abrasions and tears. Disinfectant douches are not recommended as they tend to disrupt the body's natural biological balance and destroy good bacteria as well as bad ones. For this reason, if douches are used at all, they should not be repeated more than three times a week and only plain water should be used. Douching after sex offers no protection against AIDS.

Showering immediately before sex is important because, when going to the toilet, small droplets of urine can get onto the skin around the genitals, and even though tissue paper can remove all visible faeces, tiny particles often remain. If this urine or faecal matter is infected, the HTLV–3 virus could be transmitted via body kissing of the groin and buttocks, or via touching the infected area and transferring the virus by hand to another part of the body. Though the chances of this happening are pretty slim, showering helps reduce the risk to an absolute minimum.

Lubricating from squeeze tubes or squirt-top dispensers is preferable because it prevents the supply from becoming contaminated. In contrast, lubricants such as vaseline and cold cream which come in jars can easily get infected and, by shared use, transfer the virus from one person to another. This can happen, for example, if one partner uses their finger to lubricate their anus or vagina and then inserts the same finger back into the tub to get more lubricant. If the other partner then uses the lubrication, they can become exposed to the risk of infection.

Non-penetrating sex is safest. Without penetration, it's almost impossible to exchange body fluids. So, if people don't insert parts of their body into other people's bodies, there is virtually no chance of infection. Penetrative sex, on the other hand, always involves some danger. Even in the case of mere finger penetration of the anus or vagina, this danger can be significant if the fingers are interchanged between self-penetration and the penetration of the other partner. The insertion of fingers into one body only, without interchange between partners, still carries a small risk because once they are withdrawn they can transfer infected matter to everything they subsequently touch. This risk can, however, be substantially reduced by washing immediately following withdrawal.

Penetrating oral, anal and vaginal sex with a condom is fairly safe providing the condom is used properly and both partners shower straight afterwards. Playing safely with a condom means not using an oil-based lubricant such as vaseline, body lotion, cold cream or baby oil. These cause condoms to dissolve and disintegrate. Nor is saliva a good lubricant. Apart from the possibility of transmitting infection, it is not smooth and slippery enough and therefore creates friction and tension which can cause the condom to break. It is best to use a sterile, water-soluble lubricant like KY. When rolling on a condom, leave a spare centimetre or so at the tip to allow for stretching during sex. Soon after orgasm, before the erection is lost, withdraw the penis whilst holding the open end of the condom to stop it from slipping off. In oral sex, care needs to be taken not to puncture the condom by scraping it against the teeth. And since condoms don't taste very nice, it's a good idea to add some flavouring such as honey, jam or ribena.

Playing safely ends with *showering immediately after sex*. Cleaning up afterwards is always advisable, whatever the activity, because faeces or body fluids such as semen and saliva which are left over from sex can be a potential source of infection.

Obviously, for most people, making these changes and switching to playing safely entails a major alteration in sexual lifestyle. It involves giving up, or modifying, sexual activities which people expect to do and which they are used to enjoying. It necessitates adopting new forms of sexual expression which are less familiar and, at least to begin with, probably less satisfying. To this extent, playing safely is a challenge to sexual traditions – both heterosexual and homosexual – and a challenge to each individual's sexual creativity. It impels people to rethink the nature of sexual satisfaction and the means by which it is achieved. In particular, it involves moving away from the idea that there is one form of sexual act – fucking – which is supreme and recognising that, with imagination and practice, there are many equally enjoyable routes to satisfying orgasm.

The main obstacle to the acceptance of playing safely is sexual conservatism and conditioning. Our culture is obsessed with penetration. It sees 'real sex' as consisting exclusively of penetrative intercourse – and preferably heterosexual intercourse at that! Every other form of sexual expression is relegated to the level of 'kid's stuff' or mere 'foreplay' and 'preliminaries' to the ultimate goal of penetrative orgasm. Though it is undoubtedly pleasurable, there is no physiological or psychological basis for this supposed superiority of penetrative intercourse. Indeed, not only is penetration inessential for sexual and emotional satisfaction, with the advent of artificial insemination it is now no longer even necessary for procreation! Nevertheless, the penetrative mentality is so deeply ingrained that for most people penetrative sex has become an almost automatic assumption, and often this has the rather limiting effect of reducing sex to a semi-mechanical process with only one possible end in mind.

The great virtue of playing safely is that it is different and requires people to think about what they do in bed. Instead of sex 'by rote' – a repetitive and predictable routine which begins with foreplay and invariably ends up with penetrative orgasm – safe sex involves exploration and experimentation. Far from being dull and boring, it can be very adventurous and exciting. For many people, it results in the discovery of new and immensely pleasurable dimensions of eroticism and sensuality which are ordinarily passed over in the rush to penetrative union – the multitude of erogenous zones, the diverse methods of tactile stimulation, and the sensation-heightening power of mental concentration and fantasy. Thus, whilst playing safely does mean giving up some enjoyable sexual activities, they are replaced by new ones which have their own compensatory delights and can be just as much fun.

Optimism and practice are perhaps the two most important factors in successfully and enjoyably playing safely. If people are pessimistic and think that safe sex will be boring and unsatisfying, then it probably will be. As with everything, people's expectations affect the outcome. A negative attitude tends to produce a negative experience, whilst a positive feeling is more likely to produce a positive result. And since playing safely often involves learning new sexual techniques and skills, a little practice and perseverance is required. As with anything new, safe sex rarely goes right the first time. It has to be learnt and perfected too.

If people initially feel unsatisfied and uncomfortable about playing safely, it is worth remembering that most of what we enjoy in sex is acquired and varies at different moments in our lifetime. What excites a person today might not be the same as what aroused them in previous years. At first, for example, some people find the idea of oral or anal sex a complete turn-off, yet in time it can become a favourite sexual activity. As much as anything else, therefore, playing safely is dependent on overcoming one's inhibitions and opening one's mind to new sexual possibilities. With commitment, just as we have learnt past sexual desires, so we can unlearn them and learn new ones.

If only because of force of habit, these changes in sexual lifestyle are not easy for anyone to make. But they are particularly difficult for gay men to adjust to. The homosexual community has only recently begun to emerge from centuries of savage legal repression, and many gay men are therefore understandably reluctant about giving up any of their newly won freedoms. To some, the restrictiveness of safe sex unhappily echoes the homophobia and puritanism of the New Right: witness the Conservative government's fierce defence of 'family life' and its call for a return to 'Victorian values'!

Yet in the absence of a medical cure for AIDS, it is hard to see how either gay people or heterosexuals have any real alternative.

Regrettably, the options are limited. Faced with AIDS, which threatens to decimate the gay community and gay movement if it spreads unchecked, the choice is between either playing safely or playing dangerously. Ultimately, it's a choice between survival or suicide; and the modern gay movement certainly didn't fight for sexual freedom in the 1970s so that gay men could use that freedom to commit collective suicide in the 1980s.

Choosing safe sex is thus not only a matter of individual survival, but also a question of the collective survival of the gay community and its achievements. For in this AIDS-threatened era, playing dangerously – the refusal to take care of oneself or others – is a new form of gay self-oppression. Its destructive nature embodies the unspoken message that gay people are not worth looking after and the gains of the gay struggle over the last two decades are not worth staying alive to defend and enjoy. A rather extreme view? Not really. If people value themselves so little that they are prepared to play the 'Russian roulette' of unsafe sex, then they are hardly likely to see much value in other gay people, let alone have a sense of gay pride and care about the future of the gay community. Recognising this negative and destructive nature of playing dangerously is part and parcel of the process of seeing safe sex as a positive, life-saving experience.

Perhaps one of the best plusses of playing safely is that it encourages up-front discussion about sex. Of course, safe sex can work non-verbally simply by physically steering a partner's body away from attempts at risky sexual practices towards those that are risk-free. But often a frank and open chat beforehand is the simplest and most direct way of avoiding any confusion or mistakes and ensuring that safe sex goes smoothly and with mutual satisfaction. Advance discussion of sexual expectations can also be an erotic turn-on and a great tension-reliever, creating a reassuring, trust-building and relaxing effect on both partners.

Some people, however, feel embarrassed and awkward about raising the subject of safe sex. Yet if only they knew it, probably most times their partner has the same inhibitions. Someone has to take the plunge! No one should worry if they fumble a bit with shyness. It can be quite endearing and sympathy-evoking. After all, most people appreciate sincerity far more than self-assurance and those that don't are not worth bothering with. In the small number of cases where the proposition of safe sex leads to rejection, it's probably all for the best. If a person can't respect another's wishes, and if they respect themselves so little that they are only prepared to play dangerously, then such people hardly deserve worrying about – no matter how attractive they may be!

Playing safely can, of course, be made redundant if a person feels able to enter a long-term exclusive relationship. If both partners test HTLV–3 negative after three to six months of refraining from other sexual contact and from other AIDS-risk activities such as injecting drugs, then it is fairly safe to assume that they have not been infected and can therefore do whatever they want sexually without any fear of contracting or transmitting the virus – providing they continue to maintain sexual contact exclusively with each other, or to limit encounters with other partners to 100-percent safe forms of sex such as body-to-body rubbing and mutual masturbation.

Whilst in an exclusive relationship a person loses a degree of sexual freedom, they gain the freedom of eroticism and orgasm unhindered by the constraints of playing safely. On a non-sexual level, a longer-term partner can also offer the gain of emotional support and the opportunity to develop a deeper and more meaningful association with another person which is not really possible in transitory affairs and one-off sexual experiences.

The final point on playing safely concerns sex between people who are both HTLV–3 antibody positive or who both have AIDS. It is advisable that these groups of people also follow the safe sex guidelines. This is because the HTLV–3 virus appears to mutate considerably. Picking up new and possibly more virulent strains of the virus through dangerous sexual activities could therefore cause further damage to the immune system and trigger the development of a previously dormant HTLV–3 infection into full-blown AIDS, or cause an existing case of AIDS to worsen and become fatal. This trigger effect could equally be precipitated by the transmission of venereal diseases which put the immune system under stress. In the case of two people with AIDS, the risks of unsafe sex are even greater. Not only is there the danger of passing on new strains of the HTLV–3 virus, but life-threatening opportunistic infections could also be passed from one partner to another.

Chapter 3
Fighting Back Against AIDS

The world's abloom and seems to smile,
I want to fly, but where, how high?
If in barbed wire things can bloom,
Why couldn't I? I will not die!
Concentration camp prisoner, 1944

Coping With Diagnosis

When a person is first diagnosed with AIDS, or as being HTLV–3 antibody positive, the initial reaction – sometimes immediate and sometimes delayed – is usually one of shock, anxiety and fear. Even when the diagnosis is half expected due to the presence of obvious symptoms, the confirmation of one's suspicions is still unnerving for most people. A recent AIDS patient, John, describes how he first responded to his doctor's diagnosis of Kaposi's Sarcoma: 'Panic, fear. Life would never be the same . . . Devastation . . . You have the disease that everyone fears . . . Life has turned into a nightmare of uncertainty, a bad dream with no escape.'

After a short while, the initial shock of diagnosis gives way to a flood of often conflicting feelings – disbelief, anger, depression, guilt, self-pity, despair and resignation: 'It can't be true . . . Why me? . . . I don't want to die . . . It's not fair . . . If only I hadn't . . . No one else understands what I'm going through . . . It's my own fault . . . Life's not worth living . . . Everyone can go to hell . . . I may just as well curl up and die.'

All these emotional responses are very commonplace and understandable given the gravity of AIDS and HTLV–3 infection. Indeed, it is far more healthy to be aware of and express these feelings than to bottle them up inside and refuse to acknowledge them, However, in the long term, negative and self-denigrating emotions can be very destructive. It's therefore important to find a strategy for dealing with these feelings and channelling one's emotional energies in a more outward-looking and constructive direction.

Coping with a life-threatening illness is never easy, but doing certain things can make it less difficult and enable a person to more readily overcome the trauma of HTLV–3 or AIDS diagnosis:

* Talking to other people, expressing and sharing feelings, and receiving a sympathetic hearing, can help relieve stress and reduce a person's sense of isolation and burden. As the saying goes, 'A problem shared is a problem halved.'
* Learning about AIDS and understanding it better tends to enhance a sense of self–confidence, because things always appear more frightening when we don't understand them and don't know what to expect.
* Keeping busy with activities is a useful way of preventing oneself from slipping into the kind of deep introspection and depression which can so easily take over if a person has nothing to do but sit around and worry.
* Finding and focusing on positive things which arise from diagnosis helps to render AIDS a not so wholly negative experience. The possible 'benefits' or 'advantages' of illness can include:
  – Receiving love and attention.
  – Getting closer to one's friends and rebuilding estranged relationships.
  – Being granted time off work and reduced personal responsibility.
  – Gaining an incentive to reassess one's values, reorder one's priorities and goals, and reorganise one's life.
* Looking at your troubles from a different perspective often makes them seem less of a problem and much more bearable:
  – Think of others worse off than yourself such as political prisoners suffering torture or starving children in the Third World – imagine what they are going through.
  – Look at yourself as a stranger would and try to reach a more objective and detached perception of your situation.
  – See this traumatic period in your life as being something temporary and transient.
  – Imagine yourself in ten years time looking back on these present difficulties as a thing of the past.
  – Visualise the vast expanse of the universe and just how small and insignificant your problems are by comparison.
* Drawing up a plan of action geared towards mentally and physically fighting AIDS and achieving new goals in life can

create a sense of purpose and optimism which strengthens one's abilities to cope.

These kinds of positive response to diagnosis involve a conscious intervention and assertion of self-control over one's situation. Their empowering and enabling nature can do a lot to overcome feelings of helplessness and despair. For contrary to popular perceptions, people with HTLV–3 infection and AIDS are not powerless, passive victims. They don't have to resign themselves to the 'sick role' or redefine their identity as a 'patient'. Despite infection, they can still make the positive choice to resist illness and to strive for the achievement of a happy and rewarding life.

The Will to Live

> Two things stand like stone:
> Kindness in another's trouble,
> Courage in your own.
> *Adam Lindsay Gordon, 1870*

Having the will to live is probably the most important factor of all in fighting and surviving a life-threatening condition like AIDS. Without the will to live, a person suffers more during illness, their mental and physical health deteriorates more rapidly, and death is a more certain outcome. In contrast, the determination to survive can (a) enhance the quality of a person's life during sickness, (b) extend their life expectancy beyond doctors' predictions, and (c) in some cases even lead to recovery and the resumption of a healthy and normal existence.

The fact that a person's will to live plays a significant role in the outcome of an illness has been well documented by the American cancer specialist Dr Carl Simonton, co-author of *Getting Well Again*. He discovered that cancer patients who die soon after diagnosis tend to be stricken by a sense of powerlessness and have little motivation to live. They readily give up hope, quit their jobs, withdraw from social contact with others and rapidly become apathetic, lethargic and increasingly sick. On the other hand, those cancer patients who defy the statistics by surviving against all the medical odds tend to have strong reasons for wanting to stay alive and a firm belief that they can influence the course of their illness: 'I can't die until I finish the project I'm involved with . . . They need me too much at work . . . My family could never pay off the mortgage without my income . . . I want to survive to celebrate the tenth anniversary of our relationship . . . I must heal the rift between myself and my mother before I die.' With this high degree of motivation, these patients take positive steps to increase their chances of survival and carry on living their lives as per usual for as long as they possibly can.

With AIDS, as in cancer and other life-endangering illnesses, there are four factors which are vital to create a strong and sustainable will to live – a positive mental attitude, a sense of self-esteem, a goal or purpose in life, and an active participation in fighting illness.

A Positive Mental Attitude

A person's attitude towards AIDS has a profound influence on the course of the illness. A positive expectation of recovery is likely to produce improved health, whereas a negative expectation more often results in physical and mental deterioration. This 'self-fulfilling prophecy' occurs because when people expect something to happen, they act in ways which increase the likelihood of that expectation coming true.

With AIDS, for example, if people believe that they can fight the disease, they tend to reorganise their lives around a less stressful and more healthy way of living. This often ameliorates the severity of their illness and can even lead to periods of comparatively good health – thus confirming the person's original belief and expectation. In reverse, if a person feels that they are powerless to do anything about AIDS, they tend to either live fast and wild or totally neglect themselves. When this results in declining health, it only serves to confirm and reinforce their initial feelings of helplessness.

The role of expectations in affecting the functioning of the immune system is illustrated by Dr Richard Smith's experiments at the University of Arkansas. Seven tuberculin-positive patients were inoculated in one arm with tuberculin and in the other arm with a non-reactive substance. The frequent repetition of these injections established a behavioural conditioning in which the patients expected the reaction in one arm to always be positive and the reaction in the other arm to always be negative. Then, without the patient's knowledge, the injections were switched to opposite arms. This resulted in a very drastically reduced immune reaction to the tuberculin injection – the swelling being on average only 4 mm in diameter instead of 15

41

mm. Dr Smith therefore concluded that a patient's expectation significantly affects their immune response.

In a similar vein, the way attitudes towards an illness can influence its course of development was demonstrated by Dr Simonton in his study of cancer patients at Travis Air Force base in California. He found that patients with positive attitudes had better responses to treatment, whilst those with negative attitudes had poorer responses. Even more significantly, he discovered that patients who were very seriously ill, but had positive attitudes, recovered better than patients who had less severe cancers but negative attitudes. This evidence suggests that although an optimistic and constructive mental approach may not guarantee recovery, it certainly will often lengthen life expectancy and increase the probability of survival.

In the case of AIDS – even more so than cancer – a person is confronted by overwhelmingly negative attitudes and expectations: 'Once you've got AIDS it's too late . . . There's nothing anyone can do . . . AIDS inevitably results in a rapid and painful death.' These views are not realism, but pessimism. They look at AIDS in the worst conceiveable light, and contrary to all scientific evidence deny any chance of a hopeful prognosis. Negative attitudes and expectations are thus a denial of truth and reality.

Adopting a positive mental attitude involves opening one's eyes to the possibility of taking control of the future by acting in ways which help ease suffering and prolong survival. Rather than seeing AIDS as an irreversible personal defeat and a non-commutable sentence of death, a positive response looks upon AIDS as a personal challenge which has hopeful possibilities. In the words of the Fred Astaire and Ginger Rogers musical, it means a commitment to 'pick yourself up, dust yourself down, and start all over again'.

An AIDS patient, Bill, describes how a positive mental approach helped him to survive and lead a worthwhile, enjoyable life:

> Having AIDS is not necessarily a death sentence. But judging from the statistics and how the media often reports them, a person with AIDS could understandably feel helpless, lost and resolved to an early death. Yet that is not always the case. Not every AIDS patient is gravely ill. Many are doing extremely well – living happy, productive and basically healthy lives. I am one of them. Having been diagnosed almost a year ago and having survived pneumocystis and a near fatal bout of cryptococcus meningitis, I am around to tell about it. I realise I have been lucky

and my good fortune has been through a combination of excellent health care, a great support system, and a positive attitude . . . No matter how grim the situation appears, and despite the fact that there is no cure at the moment for the disease, it is imperative to keep a positive attitude.

The value of a defiant, optimistic and constructive response to AIDS is also vouched for by Roger who has AIDS-Related Complex. He recalls the consequences of 'turning adversity into a virtue' through switching to a healthier lifestyle and radically reappraising his outlook on life:

My condition is stable and improving. Physically, I am getting a little better every month. Mentally, I am getting better every day . . . I have become a better person, with much to live for. I am doing everything in my power to get well . . . Now that I feel better about myself mentally, I'm feeling better physically.

A Sense of Self-Esteem

Having a sense of self-worth and believing in oneself enhances a positive mental attitude and the will to live. Survival is bound to be difficult unless a person is wholeheartedly convinced that they deserve to live, and unless they also have confidence in their ability to fight back against AIDS.

This means that people need to consciously reject self-denigrative and self-destructive ways of thinking. Instead, there is a need to recognise the importance of loving oneself. This is not a recommendation for vanity or egotism, but merely for people to realise that they are valuable, worthwhile individuals who deserve to be taken care of and who deserve to live a healthy and happy life. With this strong self-image and strong self-appreciation, a person is likely to fight far harder to conquer AIDS and stay alive.

In his account of a friend's battle to overcome AIDS, Christopher Spence suggests that 'self-hatred and deprecation' are two of the most formidable obstacles in the struggle against the illness. In our society, because of homophobic prejudice and discrimination, gay men face particular difficulties in overcoming guilt about their sexuality and learning to love and respect themselves. Spence identifies this lack of self-acceptance as a key factor which made his friend Frank especially vulnerable to AIDS:

When he was sixteen his Mum was killed, a loss from which he never really recovered. From then on there was always a piece of Frank which wanted to die, to be with his Mum again. He lived his life with fierce integrity but, as a working-class man, he could never recognise himself or his needs as important. As a gay man, he could not accept the reality of his deep goodness. I believe it was these three areas of deep-seated hurt, the loss of his Mum and his worthless self-image as a working-class and gay man, that made Frank so vulnerable to AIDS, and unable to combat the disease in a powerful way. It was like watching a man fight with his hands tied behind his back. A chronic feeling that you would *like* to die on the one hand, and that you *deserve* to die on the other, is hardly the best basis for resisting infection, for dealing with the terror of a life-threatening disease.

Spence concludes that

Had Frank been able much sooner to release and recover from his feelings of wanting and deserving to die – acted out in so many profoundly self-denigrating ways such as low self-esteem, low expectations and an inability to put himself first on any level -- then maybe his immune system would have been equal to the challenge of resisting the infection and he would have been able to decide wholeheartedly that he wanted to live.

A Purpose or Goal in Life

Part of the process of building a sense of self-esteem is having goals, values and priorities in life – things which make life worth living and give a person a feeling of pride and a reason for wanting to stay alive.

A serious illness like AIDS provides both a breathing space and an incentive to do things that have long been put off. It also offers an opportunity to reconsider what one wants out of life and a motive to draw up new aims and objectives. This process of setting goals and striving to achieve them has the beneficial effect of:

* Affirming your will to live and your expectation of survival.
* Giving you a motivation to fight back against AIDS.
* Expressing the self-confidence that you are in charge of your future.
* Enhancing your self-image and self-esteem as a worthwhile person with a positive contribution to life.
* Establishing a constructive focus for your energies.

Goal-setting is most helpful when the goals are concrete,

measurable and realistic, and when they are balanced between work, emotions, relaxation and health.

Work-oriented goals could include getting or changing a job, seeking promotion or an increase in salary, moving to a new house or decorating your flat, starting a project such as learning photography or a musical instrument, beginning evening classes, or involving yourself in a tenants' association, youth club, community group, political organisation or charity. Participating in organisations like Amnesty International or War on Want – which are concerned about the plight of political prisoners and hunger in the Third World – can fulfil a dual role of providing both a focus for one's emotional energies and a way of putting one's suffering into perspective. Even better, volunteer work for an AIDS information and support group like the Terrence Higgins Trust can offer a rewarding activity which simultaneously increases one's understanding of AIDS and involves a sharing of one's problems with others in the same predicament.

Emotional-oriented goals might entail rebuilding estranged relationships, overcoming guilt about one's sexuality, getting closer to family and friends or seeking a long-term partner.

Relaxation-oriented goals can consist of taking up a hobby or travel, having a regular sauna and massage, or setting aside time for movie-going, reading and listening to music.

Health-oriented goals may involve participating in a sport and doing a daily work-out, eating more nutritiously, getting regular sleep or practising safe sex.

The positive effect of this goal-setting and goal-striving is described by William, an AIDS patient who pulled through Kaposi's Sarcoma and pneumonia and went on to lead a productive life, full of achievement, for several more months:

> In the last six months, I have started my own production company, which produced a calendar of my own photography. I have worked in the community to heighten awareness of this disease. I have grown closer than ever to my family, my lover, and my friends. I am very proud and thankful for these things. Most importantly, I have come to accept myself exactly as I am. This is the greatest gift of all.

An Active Participation in Fighting Illness

Sickness is not simply something external that 'happens' to people as passive objects. People participate in the process of sickness by negative attitudes, expectations and actions; by low self-esteem and self-confidence; by lack of a purpose or motivation in life; by guilt, depression and stress; and by inadequate diet, relaxation, sleep and exercise. In all these different ways, people contribute to undermining their mental and physical defences against disease. This increases the likelihood of HTLV–3 infection developing into AIDS and decreases a person's chances of resisting and surviving the full-blown AIDS syndrome and its opportunistic infections and cancers.

However, just as people share in the process of becoming ill, they can also share in the process of getting well again. The improvement of health requires the reorientation of a person's beliefs and behaviour in a life-loving and health–affirming direction. This mobilisation of one's inner mental and physical resources in the battle against illness does more than boost bodily resistance. Participation in the process of recovery also creates a strong emotional investment in overcoming disease. This encourages a person to strive even harder in the direction of good health and gives them a measure of control and mastery over their future which is comforting, reassuring and confidence-building. Dr Arnold Hutschnecker, in his important work *The Will to Live,* argues that 'The fight against illness cannot be made by the doctor alone. The healing process must be a collaboration of both doctor and patient, a working together in the fullest sense.' A similar view is echoed by Dr Alec Forbes of the Bristol Cancer Help Centre: 'Studies have proved that when a person starts taking responsibility for his disease and reaffirming the life he possesses, he has a better survival rate that one who sits passively by.'

In the case of AIDS, given that there is no really effective medical treatment, a person's own efforts to fight the virus are especially important. This participation in the getting-well process can also be a tremendous morale booster and help ease the sense of intimidation and powerlessness which this as yet incurable disease generates. Whilst having the will to live – a positive attitude, high self-esteem, strong goals in life and an active participation in fighting AIDS – does not guarantee survival, it does shift the odds in that direction and nearly always ensures that a person survives longer and leads a more active and satisfying life while they remain alive.

Mentally Fighting AIDS

So There!

No one has told the bumble bee
That, aerodynamically,
It cannot fly
(No more can I).
So, like a furry acrobat,
It grooms its earthbound furry-fat –
Then rides the air
Bumbling, 'so there . . . !'
Kit Mouat, 1985

Health and sickness are not purely physical states of being. They are also mental and emotional states and they affect the whole person, not just their bodily functions. This interrelationship between mind, body and emotions in the causation of disease is already partly acknowledged by the medical profession through its recognition of psychosomatic illness – illness that originates with or is aggravated by a person's psychological state of mind.

From accepting that the mind can make people physically sick, it is only a short step to accept that it can also make them well again. For surely, if negative mental and emotional states can have a harmful influence on health, then positive mental and emotional states can have a beneficial effect.

In researching the personal histories of cancer patients, Dr Carl Simonton found that in the 6 to 18 months prior to diagnosis almost all of them had been through a period of intense stress, anxiety and depression which produced a sense of acute helplessness, despair and 'giving up'. These damaging emotional responses, he concluded, made the patients vulnerable to cancer, precipitating its growth and rendering them unable to fight it off.

If negative emotions could contribute to the development of cancer, Dr Simonton wondered whether positive emotions could help overcome it. Accordingly, he set up a four-year study of 159 cancer patients who were diagnosed with incurable malignancies. After training them to use their minds and emotions to fight cancer through relaxation and mental imagery techniques, Dr Simonton discovered that these patients dramatically improved their health and lengthened their anticipated survival time. By the end of the four years, 96 of the patients had died, but on average they lived for 20 months after diagnosis which is 65 percent longer than the national norm of 12 months. Of the 63 patients who were alive at the end of the study, their average survival time was 24 months – twice as long as normal – and the majority of them were almost as active and productive in their daily lives as they had been prior to the onset of cancer. Though there was new tumour growth in 20 of the 63 surviving patients, in the other 43 the cancer was either stable, regressing or had completely disappeared. These results, which were quite remarkable for a group of terminal cancer patients, convinced Dr Simonton that the mind plays 'a significant role in both *susceptibility* to disease and in *recovery* from disease . . . just as one can become psychosomatically ill, so one who is ill can move in the other direction and become psychosomatically healthy'.

The power of 'mind over matter' is not a new idea. It has been around, and proven, for centuries. Using meditation and concentration, Indian firewalkers can stride through burning hot coals without blistering their feet or experiencing any pain. Until the nineteenth century, in Europe, 'bleeding' the patient was a common and often successful treatment for disease; though in the absence of any scientific basis for this practice, its success rested almost entirely on the patient's faith in its efficacy. Amongst the Aborigines of Australia, symbolic beliefs are so powerful that the ritual of 'pointing the bone' at a person who has transgressed tribal law is sufficient to cause them sickness and death. In Africa, though the shaman's potions are some-times medicinally useless, because people believe that they have magic properties, they are usually very effective in curing ailments.

The immense power of the mind over the body is also demonstrated by the 'placebo effect'. This occurs when doctors give their patients a valueless medical preparation, such as a plain calcium pill, but inform them that it will cure their sickness – which it does – even though the preparation contains nothing of medical benefit. The only thing of value in a placebo is the patient's own belief that it will work, and it is this positive expectation alone which is so often successful in producing improved health. In a study of post-operative pain by Dr Henry Beecher and Dr Louise Lasagna of Harvard University, some patients were given morphine and other placebos. Relief from pain was reported by 52 percent of those who were given morphine and also by 40 percent of those who had the placebo. Thus the placebo was nearly as effective in relieving pain as the morphine, and this would seem to confirm that belief and expectation is a major factor in health and illness.

The influence of the mind over the body is also evidenced by biofeedback studies which have shown that it is possible for people to voluntarily control their heartbeat and other physiological reactions which were previously thought to be solely under the involuntary control of the autonomic nervous system. This technique involves attaching electrodes to the skin to monitor a bodily function like heart rate. Whenever the heart rate increases or decreases, the biological changes are fed back to the person by sounds and lights on a monitoring machine. Over time, a person learns that certain postures, breathing or thoughts can influence the heart's functioning, and by consciously repeating these they can lower or raise their heart rate virtually at will.

Using this biofeedback method, patients have been taught to modify a vast array of bodily operations, including high blood pressure, muscle tension and irregular heartbeats. This provides clear evidence that the mind can directly intervene to affect the body and its physical functioning, both for better and for worse. Biofeedback pioneers Alyce and Elmer Green of the Menninger Clinic in the United States argue that their technique proves beyond doubt that 'every change in the physiological state is accompanied by an appropriate change in the mental emotional state, conscious or unconscious; and conversely, every change in the mental emotional state, conscious or unconscious, is accompanied by an appropriate change in the physiological state'. A similar conclusion is drawn by another prominent biofeedback researcher, Dr Barbara Brown: 'Research into biofeedback is the first medically testable indication that the mind can relieve illnesses as well as create them.'

Mentally fighting back against AIDS involves the practical application of this scientific and medical knowledge using the techniques of meditation, mental imagery and positive mental reinforcement to strengthen a person's will to live, their resolve to achieve specific goals, and thereby to produce a direct improvement in their physical, mental and emotional condition.

Meditation

Stripped of its religious associations and ritual, meditation is really a very simple process of concentrating the mind. It can be used either for the affirmation of particular ideas and goals, or for the relaxation of the mind and realisation of mental peace and tranquility. In both cases – affirmation and relaxation – meditation can play an important role in countering illness.

Affirmation meditation – as outlined in Appendix 2 – involves the early morning recitation and contemplation of a poem or statement which embodies and affirms a person's will to live – their positive attitudes and expectations; their self-esteem and self-confidence; their goals in life; and their commitment to an active participation in fighting back against AIDS. It also involves a person spending time mentally setting out their concrete goals for the particular day ahead – as well as their longer-term goals for the future months – thus creating a positive frame of mind at the start of every day.

This affirmative meditation is premised on the power of mental suggestion: that positive expectations tend, in a self-fulfilling way, to produce positive results and create an uplifting sense of self-empowerment and emotional strength.

The suggestive power of the mind to effect psychological and physiological changes is demonstrated by the following simple example. When cinemas screened the film *Lawrence of Arabia,* during intermission their cafeterias reported a big increase in sales of ice-cream and cool drinks. Since the cinema temperature and the weather outside had not changed, it appears that the hot, dry desert scenes in the film had an unconscious suggestive effect on the audience which made them feel thirsty and buy more cold refreshments. Affirmation meditation works in much the same way by establishing positive mental thoughts, expectations and goals which influence a person's behaviour and physical functioning.

Relaxation meditation operates differently. Its prime purpose is to reduce stress and anxiety which undermine physical resistance to disease. Chronic stress and anxiety is always highly damaging to the body. Time and time again, medical studies have emphasised the link between stress and illness. In a pioneering investigation, Dr Thomas Holmes of the University of Washington demonstrated that personal crises such as divorce, redundancy and indebtedness nearly always precede the onset of major sickness and that the more stress people experience, the more likely they are to fall ill. His conclusion was that in situations of stress 'the activity of coping can lower resistance to disease, particularly when one's coping techniques are faulty'. Since each individual has only a limited amount of energy, if too much of that energy is directed to dealing with stress, 'we have less to spare for preventing disease. When life is too hectic, and when coping attempts fail, illness is the unhappy result.'

At the University of Montreal, Dr Hans Selye's researches suggest that chronic anxiety results in hormonal imbalances which produce physiological changes, including the suppression of the immune system. This finding has been backed up by the Australian cancer specialist, Dr Ainslie Meares. He reported that stress increases the production of cortisone and this has an inhibitory effect on the body's immune reaction.

From these studies and the vast mass of medical evidence accumulated over the last twenty years, it thus seems reasonable to assume that stress is an influence in all illness and that it is probably a contributing factor to the development of HTLV–3 infection into AIDS and to the onset of life-threatening opportunistic infections and cancers.

In these circumstances, relaxation meditation can be a helpful means of both emotionally coping with AIDS and also strengthening the body's resistance to the virus. It can be based either on fantasy or on repetitive mental exercises. Both methods achieve relaxation by blocking out distracting ideas, emotions and external stimuli and reducing all mental and physical activity to a pleasing and calming daydream or to a single simple thought – as outlined in Appendix 3.

The effectiveness of meditative relaxation in improving the health of immune-suppresed cancer patients has been well documented by Dr Ainslie Meares, a former psychiatrist and author of *The Wealth Within*. In an article in *The Practitioner* in January 1979 he reported:

In the past two and a half years, 17 patients with very advanced or terminal cancer, who have either had no orthodox medical treatment at all, or who have had cytotoxic drugs or radiation some months previously and have resumed their downhill course, have been treated in this way. Ten patients have died, but in each case their span of life far exceeded the prognosis given by experienced oncologists . . . A woman patient with an abdomen resembling a full-term pregnancy—proved at laparotomy to be due to widespread metastases—was given a prognosis of two to three weeks. With meditation she maintained an active but restricted life for 12 months . . . A man of 25 years had a mid-thigh amputation for osteogenic sarcoma and when he first saw me he already had massive secondaries in the lung, pelvis and ribs. He had dabbled in many forms of treatment, but has been constant in meditating for at least an hour a day. Now, two years and three months since my first seeing him, the bony masses on his ribs which were the size of golf balls have completely disappeared, his chest X-rays show remarkable improvement and he has just embarked on an overseas trip.

In a follow-up article in September 1982, Dr Meares confirmed his continuing success with meditation therapy and cited the following two examples:

> At surgery a woman was found to have massive involvement of the liver and other organs from carcinoma of the colon. She was advised against any attempt at chemotherapy, and her expectation of life was but a few weeks. She practised the form of intensive meditation which I have outlined, and a remarkable slowing in the rate of growth of her cancer followed. Three years later, when death was near, she looked me straight in the eyes and said, 'This has been the best six weeks of my life.' Similarly, a young woman allowed a biopsy of her breast, but refused mastectomy or chemotherapy. She practised this form of intensive meditation and now, more than two years later, she is working as a psychotherapist with a group who are helping cancer patients. She tells the patients, 'I am glad I had cancer, it has made such a change in my life for the better.'

From the success of these two women and his many other patients, Meares concluded that the meditation had enabled them 'to increase their coping ability to such an extent that they were able to face cancer without stress, with the result that their immune system was able to act more effectively on the growth'.

More recently, in an article in the *Archives of Internal Medicine* dated November 1985, Dr Richard Smith of Arkansas University has provided verifiable evidence of 'a direct link between psychological or behavourial processes and the immune system'. Once a week for nine weeks, he injected a 39-year-old woman patient with shingles virus. For the first three weeks, she was asked to produce a normal immune response, which she did. During the second three weeks, she was asked to block her body's immune response. Using meditation, she not only substantially reduced the observable skin inflammation at the site of the shingles injection, but also altered her internal lymphocyte cell activity. In the final three weeks of the experiment, the woman resumed on request a normal immune response. According to Dr Smith: 'The results from this study certainly cannot be generalised to all humans; however, perhaps other people have the ability to modulate their immune response or to develop the capacity to do so.'

Mental Imagery

Mental imagery – sometimes also known as guided imagery or visualisation therapy – is a technique which has been pioneered by Dr Carl Simonton of the Cancer Counselling and Research Center in Dallas, Texas. Premised on the power of mental suggestion to enhance psychological and physiological functioning, it involves mentally imagining the body destroying disease and becoming healthy again. The purpose of this is not self-deception or the denial of illness, but the reiteration of one's desire, and will, to get well. People who use mental imagery report feeling much more relaxed, no longer so intimidated and fearful of their illness, and invigorated with a sense of empowerment and confidence that they can, and are, playing an active role in the recovery process.

One of Dr Simonton's earliest experiments with mental imagery took place in 1971 and involved a 61-year-old man with an advanced state of severe throat cancer. He could barely swallow and was very weak and wasted, weighing only 45 kilos. Though other specialists gave him little chance of survival, Dr Simonton decided to teach the patient mental imagery. First, to breathe deeply and relax his muscles. Second, to form a mental picture of his cancer. Third, to imagine radiation therapy killing off the cancer cells. And fourth, to visualise the dead cells being flushed out of his body. Much to everyone's surprise, including Dr Simonton's, after a couple of weeks of practising this mental imagery three times a day, the patient was able to eat again and began putting on weight. Within two months, the cancer had completely disappeared. Since that initial experiment, Dr Simonton's techniques have enabled hundreds of allegedly 'incurable' cancer patients to defeat their malignancies and extend their lifespan.

Of course, mental imagery doesn't work only for cancer patients. Leon Chaitow, director of postgraduate studies at the British Naturopathic and Oestopathic Association, has reported on its successful use in the treatment of chronic teenage acne. Using mental imagery, a group of young people with severe facial blemishes who had failed to respond to any other treatment showed a dramatic improvement in their skin condition. On stopping the imagery, their acne soon returned; though those that resumed it again found that their skin cleared up once more.

For mental imagery to be successful, it is important to fulfil the following criteria:

* Repeat the imagery at least twice and preferably three times a day for a minimum of 10 minutes on each occasion.
* Prior to commencing mental imagery, get completely mentally and physically relaxed, devoid of all distractions and tensions.
* Visualise the germs and diseased cells as a defenceless enemy – small, weak, confused and easy to destroy.
* Think of the defender cells of the immune system as a powerful friend – strong, alert and readily able to destroy the illness.
* Imagine the defender cells aggressively and ferociously destroying the germs and diseased cells.
* See the germs and destroyed cells as being excreted from the body.
* Picture the damaged parts of the body as recovering and the whole body as being restored to full health.

A guide to mental imagery for people with HTLV–3 infection and AIDS is set out in Appendix 4. As indicated there, it is possible either to use realistic cell-like imagery based on the actual processes of the immune system; or to use symbolic imagery which visualises overcoming AIDS in a fantasy form as in the following two examples:

* Imagine the AIDS viruses as little hamburgers being devoured by a pack of huge, hungry dogs which represent the body's immune defenders.
* Imagine the T helper cells as an immense, teeming colony of rapidly multiplying killer bees whose vast numbers and potent stings can overpower any adversary.

These ideas for mental imagery are only illustrations. It is very important that each person experiments to discover the mental imagery which suits them best. The most effective imagery is based on letting the mind wander freely to conjure up 'spontaneous' images from deep inside the unconscious. These images reflect a person's inner, and often repressed, attitudes towards AIDS and their feelings about the possibility of recovery. Positive attitudes and feelings are more likely to produce strong and powerful images, whilst negative attitudes and feelings will tend to produce weak and impotent ones. However pessimistic, it is always better to be aware of negative attitudes and feelings, and the negative images they produce, because this enables them to be confronted and overcome.

Problems with AIDS virus imagery. If a person is deeply traumatised by the diagnosis of HTLV–3 infection or AIDS, their fear and anxiety is frequently reflected in their mental imagery. The AIDS viruses may appear as gigantic rats or dinosaurs and therefore seem very difficult to mentally destroy. One way of overcoming this problem is to picture these monster-like creatures as big inflatables and to mentally prick them with pins so they deflate and crumple into a little heap. This transforms the formerly omnipotent mental images of AIDS into one of pathetic helplessness.

In the case of realistic imagery, the problem may be that the AIDS viruses appear to be ringed by an outer wall of steel-like armour which seems to render them impregnable and impervious to destruction. This problem can be overcome by imagining acid or fire melting the protective barrier and thereby exposing the vulnerable viruses to destruction.

Problems with immune defence imagery. People's lack of confidence that they can fight back against AIDS is often reflected in their mental images of the body's defender cells. These sometimes appear small and powerless. This problem can, however, be overcome by mentally shrinking oneself to the size of a pinhead so that the defender cells seem huge by comparison; or by mentally multiplying the defender cells so that their sheer volume is so immense that they can totally swamp the AIDS viruses.

Positive Mental Reinforcement

Once a person has decided to mentally fight back against AIDS, it is essential that they surround themselves with stimuli which positively reinforce this commitment, rather than undermine it. Beautiful and inspirational influences tend to evoke cheerfulness and inner strength. Ugly and depressing influences tend to have the opposite effect. For this reason, it is important that people with AIDS should try to create an environment which reflects and stimulates their spirit of determination and hopefulness.

Redecoration. Positive mental reinforcement starts in the home. When your living situation is dark, drab and dingy, it's hard not to have negative and despondent feelings. A little redecoration, however, can brighten up even the poorest housing and make it a more pleasant place to live. Putting the effort into doing up your home is also important because it symbolises your commitment to a long-term future and your intention of staying alive to enjoy the fruits of your labour.

Redecoration need not require a great deal of work or expense:

* Repaint your home in light or bright colours.
* Put a couple of potted indoor plants and flowers in each room.
* Hang some bright new posters on the walls. Choose posters which portray the natural beauty of objects like flowers and butterflies, or which depict your idea of paradise – a tropical beach, alpine meadow, country village or desert oasis.
* Somewhere prominent in the house, display a photograph of yourself when you were at your healthiest and happiest. Look at it every day and make it your target to recapture your former mental and physical well-being.
* Also in a prominent place, pin up a drawing of your mental imagery to act as a daily reminder of your resolve to psychologically resist AIDS.

Music. Successful positive mental reinforcement can also be achieved by spending a few minutes each day, sitting quietly with your eyes closed, listening to music which is stirring and inspirational. It's a good way to start each day and put yourself in an optimistic and fighting mood. Some classical examples of inspirational music include Prokofiev's *Alexander Nevsky,* Handel's *Messiah,* Bizet's *Carmen,* Wagner's *Ride of the Valkyries,* Ravel's *Bolero,* Tchaikovsky's *1812 Overture* and Beethoven's *9th Symphony.*

Films. Another means of positive mental reinforcement is the cinema. Films whose themes focus on triumph over adversity can be a great encouragement to a person struggling against AIDS. Films like *Chariots of Fire* and *Gandhi,* for example, provide models of human will-power and courage. Likewise *Pappillon,* which recreates Henri Charrière's daring escape to freedom from the French penal colony of Devil's Island, offers an image of ingenuity and endurance in overcoming seemingly insurmountable obstacles. Even more appropriately, *Anatomy of an Illness* reenacts how the editor of the American *Saturday Review* defied medical experts by conquering an 'incurable' bone disease through a combination of positive thinking, megadoses of Vitamin C and a daily relaxation session which consisted mainly of watching lots of old Marx Brothers movies.

Books. The written word is a further source of positive mental reinforcement. Faced with a life-threatening illness like AIDS, it is often a great comfort and inspiration to read about other people who have succeeded against all the odds and to understand how they have coped with hardships and difficulties. Ludwig van Beethoven, Helen Keller, Douglas Bader and Francis Chichester, for example, each overcame disabilities and setbacks in their lives and went on to achieve great things. Other stirring examples of heroic endeavours include the following:

The Men With the Pink Triangle by Heinz Heger tells the story of a young Austrian homosexual whose iron will to live enabled him to survive five years of terror and brutalisation in the Nazi concentration camps at Sachsenhausen and Flossenburg.

Stride Towards Freedom by Martin Luther King documents the brave and dignified defiance of the Montgomery bus boycott by the Black civil rights movement which paved the way for racial desegregation in the United States.

Odette by Jerrard Tickell recounts the immense valour and perseverance of the wartime French resistance fighter and Allied agent who, despite capture and torture by the Gestapo, never broke under interrogation.

Alive – The Story of the Andes Survivors by Piers Paul Read recalls how a group of plane crash victims lost in the uninhabited and frozen wastelands of the Andes mountains never gave up hope and against all odds trekked hundreds of miles over seemingly impassable terrain to safety.

The Great Game by Leopold Trepper chronicles the courage and cunning of the Soviet spy network known as the Red Orchestra which operated clandestinely in the Nazi–occupied countries and provided vital intelligence for the Allied liberation of Europe.

The value of mentally fighting back against illness using the techniques of meditation, mental imagery and positive mental reinforcement has already been well established amongst cancer patients. Apart from Dr Carl Simonton in the United States and Dr Ainslie Meares in Australia, in Britain the self-help group Cancer Contact and Dr Alec Forbes of the Cancer Help Centre at Bristol have both had considerable success with these methods of treatment. Many of their 'terminal' cancer patients have gone on to lead normal, productive and worthwhile lives for many years after their doctors had given them up as 'hopeless' cases.

More recently, despite frequent scepticism from their medical colleagues, a few doctors in Britain and the United States have begun to adapt these methods to help people with AIDS. Dr Arnold Linken is a venereologist and psychotherapist who worked for many years at the sexually transmitted diseases clinic of Middlesex Hospital in London. Since February 1985, he has been teaching people with HTLV–3 infection and AIDS the technique of 'positive auto-hypnosis'. This involves Dr Linken hypnotising the patient and then guiding them through seven stages of mental suggestion:

1) He begins by telling the patient that they will experience relief from their symptoms of diarrhoea, fatigue, night sweats and so on.

2) He instructs the patient's unconscious that it must influence the body to get the immune system functioning properly again.

3) He asks the patient to command their T helper cells to multiply wildly like a vast field of mushrooms.

4) He calls on the patient to mentally picture themselves overcoming whatever specific opportunistic infection or cancer they are suffering from. In the case of Kaposi's Sarcoma, for example, he suggests they visualise the lesion being soothed, washed, rubbed or scratched off and that they simultaneously verbally abuse the lesion by telling it to 'fuck off' and 'burn in hell'.

5) He tells the patient to get rid of the AIDS virus from their body, either through battlefield imagery in which soldiers destroy the virus or through the patient mentally kicking or shouting it out of their body.

6) He urges the patient to view themselves in a beautiful place where they are restored to physical health and emotional happiness.

7) He concludes by reiterating each stage of the mental suggestion process.

Subsequently, the patients are taught to hypnotize themselves with the aid of a tape.

Dr Linken reports that this positive auto-hypnosis technique generally helps patients to feel 'emotionally stronger and better able to cope. They don't feel so hopeless. It gives them a more positive attitude and an improved sense of self-esteem, well-being and relaxation. Their friends and families notice the difference.'

Quite independently of any medical encouragement or supervision, other people with AIDS have begun to experiment with these alternative 'mental fightback' therapies on their own initiative. Though the numbers involved are fairly small to date, as in Dr Linken's patient group, the initial results are encouraging. Almost everyone reports feeling better in both mind and body, leading a more active life and even, in some cases, showing clinical signs of recovery.

Martin is a good example of this 'mind over matter' therapy. For 18 months he had experienced repeated bouts of opportunistic infections – herpes, thrush, CMV and a near fatal attack of meningitis. In early 1985, he began practising meditation and mental imagery using the meditative affirmation 'Every day in every way I am getting better' and using the mental imagery of soldiers in blue uniforms destroying the AIDS viruses within his body. For the last year, Martin has had no further opportunistic infections. His total white blood cell count is back to normal, his total lymphocyte count is only just below average and all the indications are that his T helper cells are on the increase again. Martin's weight has increased from 59 to 68 kilos and he now feels so 'energetic and healthy' that he is able to lead a full life, including employment in a responsible and demanding job.

Using very similar techniques, William recovered from cancer and pneumonia and went on to gain a valuable and enjoyable extra seven months of life: 'After months of medical treatment, followed by months of holistic treatment and months of spiritual work on myself, I am free. My lover's remarkable support, a spiritual guide, a meditation partner, several meditation retreats, support from wonderful friends and a lot of work within my own heart has left me at peace . . . I was given several months of relative health and energy.'

In the United States, two people with AIDS have become almost legendary for their herculean achievements in fighting back against AIDS. Tom Proctor was diagnosed with AIDS in 1984. Instead of a 'curl up and die' reaction, he decided to take up meditation and marathon running. After competing in the 1985 San Fransisco, West Hollywood and New York marathons, he was awarded a citation from his local city council for 'immense courage and compassion . . . giving hope and purpose to other people with AIDS'. Tom attributes his new-found fitness and vitality to a 'good mental attitude' and a belief that he has the 'ability to live'. Pouring scorn on the fatalists, he says: 'A lot of people think that once you get AIDS, you're bedridden and die. But if you believe you can still enjoy life and be productive, you can.'

In the first half of 1983, doctors told Louie Nasseney that he had the AIDS-induced cancer Kaposi's Sarcoma. Despite several months of treatment with the drug Interferon, his health rapidly deteriorated, the AIDS symptoms being compounded by the adverse side-effects of his medication. He suffered constant diarrhoea, fevers, headaches, weight and hair loss, hallucinations, impotence, and speech and eyesight impediments. 'I was absolutely ugly,' he recalls. Early in 1984, Louie decided to come off all drugs and begin the process of 'waking up the body, the spirit and the mind' using the 'metaphysical therapies' of meditation and mental imagery. His mental imagery was as follows: 'I imagined the lesion on my leg was a pencil mark. On the other side of a pencil is an eraser. While doing my meditation at night, I would visually erase it off my leg. It took a good six months before it started to flatten out and fade away.' To increase his depleted T helper cell population, Louie visualised them as little white rabbits: 'Little white rabbits like to multiply. That's what I needed my T cells to do. While sleeping I would visually see this happening. The immune system works at its strongest while sleeping. As of today, I have never had a higher T cell count. I have a count of 520 which is a low normal for an average person.' Simultaneously, Louie also began aerobics and weight training. Within a few months, he had built a strong, muscular physique. In late 1985 he entered the Los Angeles Super-Men muscle competition and was placed 4th runner-up – an astonishing feat for someone with AIDS! Louie attributes his recovery primarily to positive, supportive and healing thoughts:

> My metaphysical therapy has given me such a sense of well-being that I am convinced this is what saved me. I would certainly recommend this therapy to anybody, although no one can promise that it will work for a specific person. All I know is that it has worked for me.

Whilst it is impossible to tell whether Tom and Louie will remain permanently well, there is no doubt that mentally fighting back against AIDS has already given them a considerably extended lifespan and a series of remarkable personal achievements which have resulted in a profound sense of satisfaction and fulfilment.

Strengthening the Body's Physical Defences

Every day, the body produces about 100,000 cancer cells. Yet in the overwhelming majority of people these cells are naturally destroyed by the immune system, preventing them from multiplying out of control and producing tumours. Likewise, everyone is constantly exposed to cold viruses, yet we are spared permanent colds because most of the time our body's natural system of defence is able to protect against illness. Equally, only a small percentage of people with hepatitis B end up with cirrhosis of the liver. Thus, it is hardly surprising that even in the case of HTLV–3 infection, 90 percent of those affected do not get AIDS. This would seem to indicate that in some circumstances the immune system is able to effectively resist every disease, from the common cold to the most feared illnesses such as cancer and AIDS.

Why is it, then, that some people conquer disease and others succumb? In general terms, vulnerability and susceptibility to illness seem to depend to a significant degree on the state of the body's immunity. In an optimally functioning immune system, a person has a far better chance of naturally resisting all kinds of infections, including HTLV–3. On the other hand, the more a person's immune system is impaired, the worse are their chances of beating AIDS.

Immune functioning can be damaged by lots of different factors – poor diet, irregular sleep, lack of exercise, overwork, stress, depression, drug and alcohol abuse, frequent bouts of infection and so on. The cumulative effect of these immune-suppressing factors is to produce a progressively less efficient immune system which is decreasingly able to defeat illness. Recently, this view has been strongly argued by the Washington-based AIDS researcher Dr Cesar Caceres. He has suggested that HTLV–3 infection has tended to develop into AIDS amongst people whose immune systems were *already* damaged and he points to the substantially higher than average incidence of immune-suppressing recreational drug use within the AIDS-diagnosed population. Alcohol, tobacco, marijuana, poppers, cocaine and speed all depress the immune system to varifying degrees.

Dr Caceres' claims have been supported by studies at the National Jewish Center for Immunology and Respiratory Medicine which found that the use of amyl nitrate – commonly known as 'poppers' – can weaken the body's ability to fight off infections. Other researchers have also noted that a significant number of African and Haitian AIDS patients have long medical histories of repeated viral infections such as hepatitis A and B, malaria, schistosomiasis, sleeping sickness and hookworm. Furthermore, a large number of gay men with AIDS also have lengthy medical histories of frequent infection, particularly with sexually-transmitted diseases such as gonorrhea, syphilis, herpes, non-specific urethritis, proctitis and amoebic parasites.

This is not to say that previous illnesses or recreational drug use cause AIDS. They don't. However, together with other immune-suppressing factors such as stress and constant late nights, they do cumulatively undermine the immune system and thereby probably trigger, or help to trigger, the development of HTLV–3 infection into AIDS.

A person can reduce the number of AIDS 'trigger' factors by doing things which build up their immune system and avoiding things which break it down. Mentally fighting back against AIDS is one way of optimising immune functioning. Physically strengthening the body is another. It primarily involves switching to a nutritious, vitamin-fortified diet; regular exercise; and stress reduction, including plenty of relaxation and sleep. Bill, who has already adopted this 'healthy living' regime, vouches for its benefits:

> To look at me, one would never know that I have been sick or that I even have AIDS. Through a conscientious eating programme, my weight is higher now than it ever was, including before I was diagnosed. I continue going to the gym, working out every other day, which is more than most healthy persons do. I also work full-time, maintaining a basically normal workload in a productive capacity.

A Nutritious Vitamin-Fortified Diet

Everyone is familiar with the saying 'You are what you eat.' Doctors have been telling us for years that the maintenance of good health and the avoidance of disease depends in large part on a nutritionally balanced diet.

Eating the wrong foods can starve the immune system of nutrients and cause it to function under capacity. It can also cause illnesses such as heart disease and bowel cancer which wear down the body's natural defences and make them less able to cope with any subsequent infections such as HTLV–3. Conversely, eating the right foods can give the immune system a boost and shift it into top gear; thereby enabling it to attack disease wholeheartedly and with maximum potency.

Essentially, for optimal immune functioning we need to eat more natural and raw foods such as whole grains and fresh fruit and vegetables which are unprocessed and unrefined, without preservatives and other additives, and which have not been irradiated or cooked.

Many doctors are now beginning to recognise that not only is a nutritious diet essential for disease prevention, but it can also play a vital role in recovery from illness. In *Cancer and Its*

Nutritional Therapies, Dr Richard Passwater suggests that the medical treatment of serious diseases is 'doomed without proper nutrition'. He urges people to 'eat as many unprocessed foods as you can. Wash your raw foods well. Avoid foods that flagrantly pollute – especially dyed foods.'

For people with HTLV–3 infection or AIDS, the following dietary guidelines are worth considering:

More fresh fruit and vegetables. These foods contain the highest concentration of essential vitamins. Since cooking tends to destroy some of the goodness of food, the more we can eat in the raw form of salads, fruit and juices, the higher our nutritional intake. When fresh fruit and vegetables are not available, it is recommended to use frozen foods rather than tinned or dehydrated ones as the freezing process causes less vitamin destruction than canning or drying. If vegetables have to be cooked, the nutritional loss can be reduced by light undercooking, using a low heat, steaming or baking. With many vitamins being water-soluble, boiling is the most destructive method of cooking. Lost vitamins can, however, be retrieved if the cooking water is used in juices, soups and gravies. There is some evidence that aluminium damages or hinders the absorption of vitamins. For this reason, the use of aluminium saucepans and cooking utensils should be avoided in preference for stainless steel, enamel and pyrex. Given that some vitamins are destroyed if they are exposed to air or light, most fresh foods need to be stored inside dark cupboards in airtight containers or wrappings.

Less meat. Even the generally conservative medical profession now recognise that high meat consumption is a contributing factor to many diseases and have accordingly urged people to eat less of it. Apart for the high saturated-fat content of meat, modern intensive farming methods mean that animals are pumped full of hormones to stimulate their growth rates and antibiotics to keep them infection-free. Inevitably, residues of these hormones and antibiotics are ingested when people eat meat and this can have a disturbing effect on the body's hormone and immune systems. It is therefore a good idea to eat less meat and get more of our protein requirements from purer sources at the lower end of the food chain, such as fish, nuts, peas, beans, lentils, free-range eggs, cheese, soya milk and peanut butter, as well as wholemeal bread, rice and pasta.

More wholefoods. The processing and refining of food always involves discarding and destroying some of the nutrients. It also usually includes the addition of colouring, emulsifiers and preservatives which are often harmful. Indeed, many additives which have been banned on health grounds in other countries are still widely used by British farmers and food manufacturers. To avoid these dangers which put the body's digestive and immune systems under stress, and to ensure maximum nutrient content, it is advisable to eat as many wholefoods as possible, and preferably those which have been organically grown without the use of artificial fertilisers, pesticides and herbicides. Wholegrain bread, rice, pasta and breakfast cereals – plus organically grown unpeeled fruits and vegetables such as carrots and apples – are far healthier than their denatured and chemically adulterated counterparts.

Less coffee, tea and alcohol. Caffeine is an immune-inhibiting drug found in tea and coffee. These drinks, together with alcohol, tend to strain the body's immune functioning, and their intake ought therefore to be kept to a minimum by switching to decaffeinated coffee, caffeine-free herbal tea, fruit juice, milk-shakes, malted milk and drinking chocolate.

The following is a good example of a nutritionally balanced daily diet which is very easy to make and which meets the body's requirements for energy, protein, fibre, vitamins, minerals and trace elements:

Breakfast

Pure orange juice
Wholemeal muesli and milk, with mixed nuts
and diced pear, orange or banana
Poached egg topped with grated cheese, *or*
Toasted wholemeal bread with marmite or
peanut butter and honey
Herbal tea or decaffeinated coffee

Lunch

Pure carrot juice
Wholemeal bread sandwiches: Cheese, black
olives and green peppers, *or* Liver sausage,
tomato and watercress, *or* Boiled egg, tuna,
lettuce and mayonnaise
Cottage cheese with almonds or cashew nuts
and slices of apple, peach or satsuma
Milkshake made with blended chocolate,
bananas or apricots

Afternoon snack

Pure beetroot juice, *or*
Vanilla egg milkshake
Mixed nuts and raisins, *or*
Wholemeal bread sandwich made with peanut
butter and topped with mashed bananas,
walnuts and chopped dates

Dinner

Pure grape juice
Peas and sweetcorn, *or*
Shredded cabbage with slivers of dried figs
Grated carrots and roast peanuts, *or*
Diced mushrooms with spring onions
Sliced cucumber and celery sticks with blue
cheese sauce
Wholegrain rice and red kidney beans with
chopped chicken in a chili sauce
Natural 'live' yogurt with pineapple or rhubarb
and crushed ginger root

Bedtime snack

Drinking chocolate with digestive biscuits, *or*
Pure grapefruit juice with rye crispbread

People with AIDS and ARC who are experiencing significant weight loss have an additional dietary problem. To prevent themselves from wasting away, they need to dramatically increase their calorie and protein intake. The UK Recommended Daily Intake of food and nutrients suggests that just to maintain health and weight:

★ A man weighing 65 kilos, who is moderately to very active, needs a daily intake of 3,000–3,600 kilocalories and 75–90 grams of protein.
★ A woman weighing 55 kilos, who is moderately to very active, needs a daily intake of 2,200–2,500 kcals and 55–63 gms of protein.

In the case of people with AIDS and ARC, to keep their weight, skin tissue and muscle composition intact, men may need a daily intake of up to 4,500 kcals and 110 gms of protein and women may require as much as 3,500 kcals and 80 gms of protein.

These targets can be quite difficult to achieve without stuffing oneself, feeling bloated and overloading the digestive system. There are several solutions to this problem:

* Add lots of high-calorie dressings, sauces, garnishes and toppings to food – polyunsaturated magarine, pickle, yogurt, mayonnaise, gherkins, chutney, tomato sauce, mustard, salad cream, peanut butter, desiccated coconut, and sachet sauces such as chili con carne and cauliflower cheese.
* Drink most of the body's liquid intake in the form of high-calorie chocolate milkshakes, hot drinking chocolate, fruit juice fortified with dried skimmed milk, or prepackaged energy supplements such as Complan and Enrich.
* Eat between meals high-calorie snacks like chocolate, potato crisps, biscuits and fruit cake.
* Instead of having three huge meals a day, try to eat four slightly smaller ones.

Just as calories are necessary for energy, activity and weight maintenance, protein – the building block of life and the essential constituent of all cells – is vital for the repair and growth of the body, especially during illness when it is subject to stress and damage. The most dense sources of protein are soya beans and milk, cheddar cheese, roast peanuts, marmite, prawns, turkey, peanut butter, red kidney beans, fish, chicken, liver, bacon, pork, lamb, muesli and eggs.

For people with AIDS and ARC who are trying to maintain or regain their weight by increasing their calorie and protein intake, it's important not to overeat and end up becoming overweight. The volume of calories and protein should only be increased to the extent that they are necessary to keep a healthy weight level relative to a person's height. Whilst increasing the calorie and protein content of the diet, it's also essential to get plenty of exercise to ensure that the extra calories and protein are converted into muscle and skin tissue, rather than being deposited as fat. People who experience a difficulty in eating due to loss of appetite might find it helpful to stimulate the appetite acupressure point on the fourth finger, as indicated in Appendix 9.

The treatment of disease using nutrition supplements in the form of megadoses of vitamins and minerals is still regarded as highly dubious in conventional medical circles – even though there is a growing volume of scientific evidence which points to their efficacy. Interest primarily focuses on vitamins A and C and the minerals zinc and selenium, each of which seem to have at least some immune-boosting capacity when tested out on cancer patients.

Nobel Prize winner Dr Linus Pauling has for many years argued that vitamin C can significantly contribute to the prevention and cure of many diseases – including the common cold and cancer – by 'bolstering the body's natural protective mechanisms'. His colleague and co-author of *Cancer and Vitamin C*, Dr Ewan Cameron, has conducted a number of clinical trials at the Vale of Levan Hospital in Scotland using vitamin C to treat terminally ill cancer patients. After injecting patients with 20 grams of vitamin C a day for ten days, followed by an oral dose of 10 grams daily, Dr Cameron found a general improvement in the health of all patients and spectacular recovery in a few cases.

These results, which have been reconfirmed in repeated trials since the early 1970s, have been backed up by Dr Richard Passwater in the United States. He has reported that breast cancer patients treated with vitamin C lived six times longer than a matched control group, while kidney patients lived five times longer. Recent studies in Japan have also indicated that 20 gram intravenous doses of vitamin C can directly inactivate some viruses.

An article in the *Lancet* on 11 August 1984 presented evidence that vitamin A 'profoundly influences the regulation of cell proliferation and differentiation, and can inhibit tumour development'. Drawing on scientific studies over the last six years, the author pointed out that the retinol form of vitamin A and its associated retinoids have variously been shown to suppress the malignant transformation of cells exposed to chemical carcinogens; alter cellular growth factors; sometimes halt the proliferation of cancerous invasive cells; and cause active cancer cells to become non-malignant. The article cited the fact that low blood retinol levels have been found to correlate with a subsequently increased incidence of lung cancer. Conversely, twenty different retrospective studies have shown that above-average intake of the other form of vitamin A, beta-carotene, consistently results in a lower than average incidence of cancer. These findings led the *Lancet* to propose that vitamin A may well help to prevent the development of carcinomas. However, when it came to the curative value of vitamin A, the *Lancet* was less hopeful. After evaluating clinical trials using various retinoids, it concluded that the regression rate has been fairly small, though with some specific types of cancer retinoid treatment has produced significant improvements. In patients with superficial bladder papillomas, for example, the prescription of oral etretinate has resulted in a substantially lower incidence of recurrences than amongst patients given a placebo in a double-blind randomised trial.

Dr Richard Passwater and Dr Hans Nieper have suggested that zinc can assist the activation of the immune system by stimulating the development of new T cells and increasing their overall numbers, especially when it is taken in conjunction with vitamin A. In July 1983, the *Lancet* reported that a regular intake of selenium is a possible factor in the prevention of cancer and an American survey found that people eating a selenium-deficient diet were six times more likely to develop cancer than those with an adequate selenium intake.

The value of vitamin therapy is strongly defended by Dr Alec Forbes of the Cancer Help Centre in Bristol. In addition to a diet based on raw fresh wholefoods, for strengthening the body's immunity he prescribes supplements of vitamin C, vitamin A in the form of pure carrot juice, zinc, selenium, magnesium, ginseng, vitamin D2, vitamin E and the whole vitamin B complex.

Following a similar regime of megavitamin therapy, Maurice Burke overcame a cancer which conventional medical treatments were unable to cure. In 1976, he started developing a mysterious swelling in his neck. Two years later, baffled doctors advised a biopsy and an apple-sized cancerous mass was subsequently removed by surgery. Thereafter, he underwent chemotherapy and radiotherapy. However this treatment caused appalling side-effects, making him feel worse than ever and rendering him barely mobile. What is more, it failed to stop the tumour from regrowing. Losing all faith in conventional medicine and facing the possibility of imminent death, Burke turned in desperation to the alternative holistic medical ideas published in the American journal *Prevention*. On reading an article about Dr Ewan Cameron's experiments with vitamin C, he arranged for a sympathetic doctor to administer daily 20-gram intravenous injections. He recalls: 'Nothing happened for the first four days but, on the fifth day, Friday, while the vitamin C was being administered, I began to feel better. I mean I was now suddenly feeling like it was nice to be alive. I had not felt that way for months.'

After nine days, Burke discontinued the injections as the repeated large intravenous doses were having an adverse effect on the veins in his arms. Instead, he switched to taking 16 grams a day orally. Soon afterwards, he read of a report from the National Institute of Health in Washington that megadoses of vitamin A had been clinically shown to produce beneficial results in cancer patients. So Burke took 50,000 iu's of vitamin A daily – half in the form of fish oil and half in the form of beta-carotene. Simultaneously, on reading about the immune-boosting effects of the mineral selenium, he added 300 mcg. in its organic seleno-amino acid form to his daily vitamin regime. Burke began to feel more and more healthy. Then, six weeks after starting the vitamin C therapy, his neck suddenly swelled up enormously. Burke was devastated. Concluding that the cancer was spreading out of control, he mentally prepared himself for the worst. Much to his surprise, three weeks later the swelling began to recede. Within two months it had completely disappeared and he was able to resume his demand-ing job as an international industrial designer. Subsequent medical tests confirmed that Burke had no trace of cancer.

When it comes to people with HTLV–3 and AIDS, the value of megavitamin therapy is difficult to assess. However, on balance, given that it has shown some effectiveness against other serious diseases like cancer, large vitamin doses are probably worth trying. They certainly cannot do any harm and may well do some good. The following daily doses could be helpful:

* *Vitamin C: 6 grams* – 2 grams three times a day, preferably in the form of calcium ascorbate.
* *Vitamin A: 30,000 iu's* – half in the form of fish oil and half in the form of beta-carotene.
* *Selenium: 200 mcg.* – taken in the form of organically bound seleno-amino acid.
* *Zinc: 50 mg.*

People with ARC or AIDS who are currently experiencing severe ill-health, including opportunistic infections or cancers, could consider even larger doses of vitamin C – 10 grams a day – though the dosage should be reduced if it causes diarrhoea. It is advisable that vitamin C be taken after a meal or snack with a glass of milk. This is because large intakes can cause mild intestinal upsets if ingested on an empty stomach. Since vitamin C dissipates the body's calcium content, milk is important to maintain adequate calcium levels. It can also help to neutralise the acidity of large vitamin C doses. People who are allergic to milk can replace lost calcium by increasing their intake of other calcium-concentrated foods such as watercress, beans, dried figs, almonds, muesli, pilchards or sardines. In the case of vitamin A, it is important that the dosage is split into fish oil and beta-carotene forms, partly because they act in slightly different ways and partly because beta-carotene can be toxic in very high doses. As a general guide, for safety's sake, total vitamin A intake in tablet and food forms should remain well below 100,000 iu's a day. Anyone deciding to try this vitamin therapy should inform their doctor as it may have an effect on the results of clinical tests. All the above-mentioned vitamins and minerals are available in chemists or health food shops.

A final therapy which may be useful is Iscador, a medicinal extract of mistletoe which has been used, with some success, as a treatment for cancer. In *The Cell, the Human Organism and Cancer*, Dr Rita Leroi points out that Iscador has been shown experimentally to stimulate the thymus gland which gives rise to the T cells of the immune system, increasing the numbers of T cells and also the numbers of granulocyte scavenger cells. Currently, Iscador injections are being used as part of Dr Alec Forbes' treatment programme at the Cancer Help Centre in Bristol.

Plenty of Exercise

The value of regular exercise in promoting good health has long been medically recognised. A strong fit body is far better able to resist infection than a weak, run-down one. The virtues of exercise are:

* Physically, it oxygenates the blood, improves circulation, removes body toxins through the sweat glands, massages the internal organs, and stimulates the functioning of the immune system by releasing more activated white cells into the blood-stream.
* Psychologically, it relieves stress and tension and creates positive feelings of vitality, health and well-being. In Norway, controlled studies by Dr Egil Martinsen have demonstrated that frequent exercise can help alleviate depression.

For people in relatively good health, Appendix 5 sets out a daily early morning work-out programme designed to exercise all the main muscle groups in the body. In adition, it's probably a good idea to try to get an hour's intensive hard exercise once a week through an activity like squash, tennis, gymnastics, judo, weight training, football, jogging or vigorous disco dancing, swimming or cycling. People who do regular exercise should remember that it is important to have a diet adequate in calories and protein to sustain muscle tissue and replace the energy burnt up in exercise; otherwise they will tend to lose weight and develop feelings of tiredness and exhaustion.

For people who are seriously ill with ARC or AIDS, but still mobile, a more gentle start to exercise is recommended:

★ Begin with short walks to the shops or to a friend's home. As you gather strength, gradually lengthen the walks and increase their frequency. Try climbing up and down flights of stairs.
★ Progress to leisurely bicycle rides, walks interspersed with bursts of jogging, short swimming sessions and a little disco dancing.
★ Once you feel comfortable with these exercises, move on to the warm-ups in the work-out guide. When the warm-ups start to feel not too much of a strain, attempt the work-out itself.

For people who are bedridden with ARC and AIDS, it is advisable to start with:

★ Mental imagery – visualise yourself exercising and gaining strength and health.
★ Thereafter, try the following bed-based exercises – raise and lower arms and legs; clench and relax leg muscles; point and unpoint toes; open and close fists; and roll the head and the neck.
★ Then, as you feel stronger, take short walks around the room and do some exercises which involve bending down and raising your hands above your head.
★ Having accomplished this, try climbing up and down a short flight of stairs or repeatedly sitting down and standing up again.

Regular Sleep

The basic function of sleep seems to be one of mental and physical rejuvenation. As we sleep, our minds and bodies are able to rest and recharge their energy levels whilst at the same time performing operations which are essential to our well-being: the brain processes and files the information it has received during the day and the immune system is able to function at its maximum efficiency because it is subject to less psychological and physical stress during our non-waking hours. Thus, getting adequate sleep is part and parcel of the process of maintaining good health and overcoming illness. Without it, we end up feeling tired, confused, run down and prone to colds, flu and other infections.

The amount of sleep a person needs can vary quite widely from one individual to another. Whilst some people need a solid eight hours a night, others seem to get by adequately on six or seven. It's therefore not possible to lay down any hard and fast rule beyond the recommendation that each person should aim to get enough sleep so that on waking up in the morning they feel relaxed, refreshed and ready for an energetic day's activity. Waking up in the morning and feeling tired, headached, tense or reluctant to get out of bed is a sign of inadequate or unrelaxed sleep – and probably an indication of stress and emotional upset as well. Faced with these warning signs, a person needs to aim for either longer, deeper or more tranquil patterns of sleep.

As a general guideline, someone with HTLV–3 infection should try to get about eight hours sleep a night. People with PGL, ARC and AIDS who are very fatigued may need an additional afternoon or early evening nap. It is important to avoid losing sleep for more than one night in succession. A late night should be followed by an early one to make up for lost sleep.

A deep and relaxed sleep requires:

* A comfortable warm bed, preferably with a firm mattress to ensure a good sleeping posture.
* A dark, quiet room. If your bed is currently in a part of the house which is prone to noise disturbance, perhaps you ought to consider moving it to a quieter room.
* A well ventilated bedroom. In a small confined room without enough fresh air to breathe, the brain can become starved of oxygen and this causes headaches and grogginess (overheating a bedroom can produce similar effects).
* A state of mental and physical relaxation. Anxiety and tension tend to result in sleeplessness and nightmares. These problems can be alleviated by the following pre-bed relaxation techniques – listening to soothing music, being body massaged, taking a warm bath, doing relaxation exercises or

relaxation meditation, having a hot drink and sex or masturbation. Once in bed, if you still have trouble sleeping, try the relaxation meditation technique of stilling your mind by thinking of a totally black space or by visualising a beautiful and tranquil scene.

Stress Reduction

More and more doctors now accept that stress plays a significant role in the onset of disease and that relief from stress can aid recovery from illness.

On 20 July 1985, the *Lancet* presented a summary of recent clinical studies which have drawn direct correlations between the incidence of stress, suppressed immunity and the subsequent development of sickness. It suggested that these studies demonstrate that stress can 'modify the immunologic mechanisms of the host and alter the course of infection and disease'. This realisation has given birth to a new interdisciplinary science known as 'psycho-immunology'. Broadly speaking, it is premised on the proposition that stress produces direct physiological changes such as increased secretion of cortico-steroid hormones which suppress the production or activity of the immune system's white blood cells whose function is to seek out and destroy infections.

The *Lancet* article begins by referring to the 1977 study by Dr R. Bartrop at the University of New South Wales in Australia. Comparing bereaved and non-bereaved persons, he found that the stress of bereavement substantially lowered the body's immune response. In particular, it depressed the reaction of the key white blood cells, the T lymphocytes. In the United States in 1983, Dr S. Schleifer's experimental trials with different categories of hospital inpatients and outpatients reported a clear link between severe depression and subnormal T lymphocyte activity. A seventeen-year study of 2,020 middle-aged men by Shekelle (1981) found that those who showed signs of depression at the beginning of the study had a subsequent cancer death rate twice as great as persons whose tests revealed non-depressed psychological states. Meyer and Haggerty's (1962) examination of the case histories of sixteen American families discovered that chronic stress correlated with increases in streptococcal infection. The clinical observation of military cadets by Kasl (1979) indicated that those experiencing intense academic pressure were more likely than others to contract infectious glandular fever. The *Lancet* article concludes by referring to Baker and

73

Brewerton (1981), who found a recurrent pattern of increased stress in the months before the onset of acute rheumatoid arthritis in women.

These findings have been reconfirmed in even more recent studies. In 1986, Professor Cary Cooper of the University of Manchester Institute of Science and Technology completed a four-year study of 2,163 women screened for breast cancer. He discovered a definite statistical link between the development of breast cancer, the experience of stress and an individual's inability to cope with it. Likewise, after a ten-year study of 1,000 people in a small Yugoslav town, Dr R. Grossarth-Maticek came to a similar conclusion: that the number of traumatic life events evoking a sense of chronic helplessness was a strong predicator of a person's probability of contracting cancer. This is not to suggest that stress causes cancer, or any other disease, but that it *does* suppress the immune system and thereby allow illness to develop.

Given so many cases of clear medical evidence that stress is linked to many different illnesses, it seems reasonable to assume that it is also probably a factor in the development of HTLV–3 infection into AIDS and in the onset of life-threatening opportunistic infections and cancers. If you are at risk, it is therefore sensible to take steps to reduce your stress level. This can be done by (a) avoiding anxiety-provoking situations, (b) pacing yourself and not taking on too many responsibilities, (c) expressing your emotions rather than bottling them up inside, (d) overcoming present and past emotional traumas which have produced stressful feelings of resentment, loss, guilt and rejection, (e) seeking the emotional support of a counsellor or 'buddy' partner who also has HTLV–3 infection or AIDS, and (f) practising techniques of mental and physical relaxation.

Stress reduction first involves recognising the warning signs of anxiety:

Physical signs of stress include headaches, diarrhoea, sweating, indigestion, sleeplessness, neck and back tension, accelerated heartbeat and breathing, nail biting, eye strain, skin rashes, trembling, nausea, clenched hands, loss of appetite, overeating, fiddling with hair and clothes, licking and biting lips, and increased sensitivity to noise, touch and bright lights.

Psychological signs of stress include nervousness, worry, depression, bad temper, forgetfulness, indecision, irritability, moodiness, impatience, confusion, restlessness, and lack of concentration.

The presence of two or more of these signs can very often be an indication of stress and a signal that, for the sake of your health, you need to take action to alleviate the tension and anxiety. Roger, who suffers from ARC, has noted a substantial improvement in his condition since he started taking positive action towards reducing the stresses in his life:

> I had to change my attitude towards stress. Stress is not something that has to come with life in the big city or running a business. Stress is the result of trying to do too much, poor scheduling, and a desperate need to be so busy that you don't think. Stress comes from not handling situations in a mature and rational manner . . . It is important that I surround myself with people who avoid stress, not produce stress . . . I have learned that I have to schedule a nap every afternoon in order to have good energy for the rest of the day. I have to pace myself and not take on too much responsibility or too many obligations. My health is the most important thing.

There are many different and often very pleasurable ways in which people can relieve stress and learn to unwind and relax:

* *Deep breathing*. Taking long, slow, deep breaths for a couple of minutes is a very simple way of calming oneself. It's the sort of thing you can do almost anywhere at any time – on a train, in a queue, at a meeting or during work. See Appendix 5.
* *Relaxation meditation*. This technique, as set out in Appendix 3, is an excellent means of creating a sense of mental stillness and tranquility. It also indirectly helps to ease physical symptoms of anxiety such as 'butterflies' and palpitations.
* *Relaxation exercises*. Stress frequently produces muscle tension which in turn can cause headaches. The gentle physical exercises in Appendix 6 are designed to unwind and stretch the muscles to produce a feeling of deep bodily relaxation.
* *Work-out*. A vigorous physical work-out, as illustrated in Appendix 5, helps dissipate anxiety and the energy which anxiety thrives upon. It leaves the body pleasantly tired and ready for rest.
* *Body massage*. The most enjoyable and sensual method of physical relaxation is massage. Appendix 8 gives a guide to basic massage techniques for the easing of muscle tension and the assurance of a good night's sleep.
* *Turkish bath or sauna*. Many people find a weekly turkish bath or sauna is an effective way of unwinding and sweating out the body toxins; especially when it is combined with a body

massage and swim.

* *Acupressure*. This method for relaxation and the treatment of minor ailments is based on the principles of the ancient Chinese practice of acupuncture. According to these principles, there are twelve meridians of energy which flow through the body. When these get blocked or damaged, stress, pain and illness occur. Thus, by manipulating certain points on the body – usually around bundles of nerves or nerve junctions – pain can be relieved and relaxation and health restored. Acupressure uses the same meridians and points as acupuncture. But instead of inserting needles, finger and thumb pressure is applied, as indicated in Appendix 9. Though acupuncture and acupressure undoubtedly are of medical benefit, they are still not very well understood scientifically. Some recent studies have, however, given these methods an increasing scientific foundation. It has been shown, for example, that acupressure stimulation of certain parts of the body releases pain-killing endomorphins. These long chains of peptides produced by the pituitary gland have a similar effect to morphine in deadening pain.

* *Reflexology*. Related to the theories of acupuncture and acupressure, reflexology is based on the hypothesis that channels of energy run vertically through the body and end up in the feet; and that each organ and muscle in the body is connected through a network of nerves to a particular part of the feet. In other words, reflexes in a person's feet are linked to reflexes in the rest of their body. Thus, by thumb pressure at a specific point on the foot, reflex reactions can be stimulated at a specific point in the body. This stimulation has the effect of improving physical functioning and promoting relaxation. Though there is very little scientific evidence to substantiate the theory of reflexology, it certainly does seem capable of inducing a heightened state of physical relaxation. The reflexology relaxation method involves thumb pressure massage all over the foot, moving each toe in small circular motions, rubbing the foot vigorously between both hands to create heat, rotating the foot on the ankle, firmly squeezing the foot between the palms, stretching each toe lengthways, and downward pressure between the toes.

* *Qi Gong*. Another acupuncture-related therapy is Qi Gong self-massage – pronounced 'chee gong' – a few examples of which are depicted in Appendix 7. Over 3,000 years old, Qi Gong is ideal for overcoming tiredness and tension to produce feelings of refreshment and invigoration.

* *Yoga*. Yoga includes different mental and physical disciplines. Hatha Yoga is the discipline which deals specifically with the body. Whereas weight training involves muscle contraction, Hatha Yoga consists of muscle extension. This is achieved through a set of slow, rigorous, controlled and harmonious movements. Their objective is to realise certain specific postures known as 'asanas'. To realise the Mudra asana, for example, you need to sit erect and cross-legged on the floor with your arms clasped across your chest. Take a deep breath. Then breathe out and bend slowly forward till your forehead touches the floor. Hold this position for as long as feels comfortable. The effect of Hatha Yoga is to stretch the muscles and, like a big yawn for the whole body, produce a sense of relaxation, flexibility and suppleness.

* *Music*. Soothing music can be a very serene method of relaxation. Some good examples of relaxing classical music include: the prelude to Wagner's *Tristan and Isolde*, Debussy's *La Mer*, the slow movement from Beethoven's *Moonlight Sonata*, Delius' *Brigg Fair*, Handel's *Water Music*, Mendelssohn's *Fingal's Cave* (from the *Hebrides Overture*), Bach's *Air for the G String*, the Prelude to Verdi's *La Traviata*, Sibelius' *The Swan of Tuonela* and Ravel's *Pavane Pour Une Infante Defunte* and *Lever du Jour*.

* *Laughter*. Perhaps the best 'medicine' of all, laughter is one of the simplest and most effective relaxation therapies. Furthermore, by putting a person in a happy unstressed state of mind, laughter can actually enhance the functioning of the immune system. It is also excellent exercise for the muscles of the face and the abdomen and its internal massage effect helps to stimulate glandular and digestive activity. People with HTLV–3 infection or AIDS will therefore find that it buoys up both their spirits and their health if they can get at least half an hour of laughter every day from newspaper cartoon strips, joke books, comedy films, records, radio shows or television series. Most local libraries carry a selection of records by comedians such as Jasper Carrot, Joan Rivers, Tony Hancock, Spike Milligan, the Two Ronnies, Flanders and Swann, and Peter Cook and Dudley Moore. Nearly every night there are at least two or three comedy series on television – *Yes, Prime Minister, Spitting Image, Brothers* and *Cheers* to name just a few. There are also plenty of comedy films by stars like Woody Allen, Peter Sellers and John Cleese; plus the classics – the Marx Brothers, Laurel and Hardy, Charlie Chaplin, the Three Stooges, W.C. Fields and Buster Keaton.

* *Sunlight*. Everyone knows how relaxing and calming it is to sit in warm sunlight. The sun's rays are also a primary source of vitamin D and help increase the production of phosphorous, calcium and iron in the blood.

HTLV–3 and AIDS Support Groups

The diagnosis of HTLV–3 infection or AIDS often leads to a profound sense of isolation. Sometimes this is self-imposed through feelings of guilt, regret, worthlessness and a belief that no one else can ever adequately appreciate the emotional trauma and physical suffering induced by AIDS. Other times, the isolation is socially enforced through the often irrational fear and hysteria which AIDS has generated in the public mind. This can lead either to outright rejection by family, friends and work colleagues, or to a more subtle and silent avoidance in which former associates keep their distance or lose direct contact altogether. If a person's AIDS status becomes more widely known, it can also prompt cruel discrimination and ostracism by neighbours, local shops and even by hospital staff. In all cases, the resulting isolation is very demoralising and destructive, producing intense feelings of loneliness and embattlement at precisely the moment when social contact and emotional support is most vital.

Overcoming isolation and securing emotional succour are critical components in the fightback against AIDS. Very few people can face serious illness alone. To admit this is no shame and no measure of personal inadequacy. Even at the best of times, we all need emotional support from other people. In the case of AIDS, the need is simply greater than normal. If a person has a supportive lover or family, then they are probably able to satisfy most of their emotional needs and receive sufficient encouragement in their resistance to AIDS. However, for those without lovers, or whose family have rejected them because they are gay, getting adequate emotional satisfaction and sustenance in their struggle against illness is much more difficult. For these people, in particular, it is imperative that they find some way of receiving sympathetic understanding, encouragement and reinforcement.

One way of achieving this emotional comfort and overcoming isolation is through the network of AIDS support and self-help groups which have sprung up over the last couple of years. Britain's main AIDS charity, the Terrence Higgins Trust, organises groups for people with AIDS and Body Positive organises groups for people diagnosed with HTLV–3 infection. Both these organisations provide the means by which people can meet others in the same predicament and share their feelings and problems. These organisations are also valuable because many people find it easier to start the fightback against AIDS, and make the radical changes in their lifestyle which are necessary, if they have the support and encouragement of a 'buddy', or companion, who is in the same situation. The empathy and mutual positive reinforcement which one can give the other is a tonic in itself – especially for those without lovers, and all the more so in such cases if it can subsequently develop into a deeper loving relationship. For even in the midst of struggling for their lives, partnerless people infected with the HTLV–3 virus should not close their mind to the possibility of building a rewarding relationship. Indeed, for some people, it can be their emotional and physical salvation.

Chapter 4
Living with AIDS

> To live badly is not to live,
> But to spend a long time dying.
> *Democritus of Abdera, circa 420 B.C.*

Self-Care and Home Hygiene

For some people, their inclination on being told of HTLV–3 diagnosis or on falling ill with AIDS is to adopt a fatalistic attitude, lose all hope, and cease to bother about anyone or anything. They start to take less care of their appearance and allow their home to fall into a state of untidiness and chaos. Once people let themselves go like this, they tend to very quickly get locked into an accelerating downward spiral of apathy and self-neglect. Quite literally, this is a fatal mistake – a sure recipe for rapid mental and physical deterioration.

Critical to a person's survival is the maintenance of a sense of dignity and self-esteem. This means, despite illness, making the effort to look after oneself and one's home. It means striving to sustain an attractive appearance and pleasant living environment. This is often very difficult for those who are seriously ill with ARC or AIDS. Nevertheless, even then it is important for a person's feelings of self-worth that they at least try as best they can.

With the diagnosis of HTLV–3 infection, a person doesn't cease to be safe to live with or to visit. Avoiding the transmission of infection to others in the home simply means that new rules of living need to be learnt and new precautions need to be taken. They may seem a bit tiresome at first. If, however, they can protect your health and the health of those who live with and care for you, then a few basic 'do's' and 'don't's' are well worth the effort. This maintenance of personal and home hygiene is not only healthy, it also has the beneficial psychological effect of making you feel better and reassuring anxious friends so that they feel happy to be around you.

* Lots of infectious micro-organisms accumulate on the skin. Some of these can potentially cause infections. It's therefore important to bathe or shower daily, using plenty of soap and rinsing the body thoroughly to carry away any germs and dirt. It's advisable to keep your own separate soap and towel, rather than sharing. Liquid soap dispensers are safest because, unlike bars of soap, the source cannot become contaminated with infected body fluids.
* If you use an enema or douche, keep it to yourself and don't loan it to others. In the case of a reusable douche set, always wash it in hot soapy water after each use.
* The gums are very sensitive and can easily by damaged by toothbrushes, dental floss and toothpicks. These should therefore be used gently and never shared with other people.
* Since fingernails and toenails can harbour germs, it's a good idea to keep them clipped short and to daily scrub them with a nail-brush.
* Any cuts or scratches on the body should be covered with a waterproof plaster till they are healed.
* Used tissues, tampons and dressings are most safely disposed of down the toilet.
* Razors ought not to be shared because they often cause minor cuts and get contaminated with particles of blood. The risk of cuts can be reduced by using an electric razor instead of a wet-shave blade.
* After going to the toilet, always thoroughly wash your hands in hot soapy water.
* In the event of spilling blood, vomit, saliva, nasal fluid, tears, vaginal secretions, urine, semen or faeces on your body, or on someone else's, you should:
    – clean it up with tissues and then flush the tissues down the toilet;
    – wash the affected skin area, preferably with a strong anti-viral and anti-bacteriological soap like Betadine Cleanser or Hibbiscrub;
    – wipe the floor and any other affected household surfaces with a 1 in 10 dilution of Domestos bleach.

If you need help to clean up spilt body fluid, the other person ought to wear household rubber gloves in case their skin is damaged and the virus gets into their blood via a crack or graze.

* To protect your body from germs, the toilet, bath, shower and wash-basin should be twice weekly disinfected with a solution of 1 part of bleach to 10 parts of water. This concentration is capable of destroying most germs, including the HTLV–3 virus.

Kitchen care

* Always wash your hands thoroughly in hot soapy water before preparing food and before eating. If you have any scratches or cuts on your hands, in addition to covering them with waterproof plasters, it might be a sensible extra precaution to wear a pair of rubber gloves when cooking – though *not* the same pair that you use to wipe up body spills!
* Scrub all raw foods well with a vegetable brush.
* Make sure all meat and seafood is properly defrosted, well cooked and that any leftovers are kept refrigerated, never reheated and eaten within three days.
* Avoid the temptation to dip your fingers into the food to taste it as you cook.
* Keep the inside of the bread-box, vegetable rack and refrigerator clean and mould-free by frequently clearing out old, stale food and by washing them regularly with hot soapy water containing 10 percent bleach.
* After meals, wash all dishes and utensils in detergent and water hot enough to need gloves.
* Don't use kitchen cleaning cloths in the bathroom or the toilet, or vice versa. Keep them separate.
* Never pour water used for cleaning the floor or the toilet/bathroom down the kitchen sink where food is prepared and where dishes are washed.

Laundry care

* Ordinarily, clothes can be safely cleaned using the hot wash cycle of a washing machine.
* Clothing or bed linen that has been badly soiled with body fluids can either be boiled or soaked in bleach in accordance with the recommended dilutions on the product label. However, this is not essential and simply ironing your laundry after a hot wash is probably just as effective. Care should be taken *not* to boil, bleach or overheat the iron on delicate fabrics.

* Since pets can sometimes carry opportunistic infections such as Toxoplasmosis Gondii, it's worthwhile getting them checked by a vet and treated for any potentially communicable diseases.
* When cleaning animal spills, litter boxes, aquariums or bird cages, always wear rubber gloves.
* In the case of cat and bird trays, at least once a week disinfect them with 1 in 10 dilution of bleach and dispose of their litter in tied bin-liners.
* Because parasites and other infections are transmissable through raw flesh, it is best only to feed your pet cooked meat.
* Pets that are exclusively indoor animals and have no contact with other animals outside the house pose the least risk of passing on disease.
* Keeping pets is safe if you follow these guidelines. Don't panic and get rid of them. Especially if you live alone, having a pet can be a great source of companionship, emotional comfort and relaxation. As studies of the elderly and housebound have shown, the simple act of nursing and stroking a cat seems to reduce stress and induce a sense of calm and tranquility.

Sustaining Sexual Relationships

People facing a life-threatening illness like AIDS have a stronger than ever need for emotional expression, closeness, warmth, tenderness and the reassurance that they are still loved and desirable. Sustaining or building a relationship during the crisis of AIDS can therefore be a pivotal part of the healing process; providing emotional support, enhancing self-valuation and precipitating inner psychological strength. Conversely, the sudden axing of an existing relationship can provoke profound trauma, self-doubt and stress which make it all the more difficult for the person to mentally and physically resist illness.

People infected with HTLV–3 are understandably anxious about passing the virus to others. However, even if their partner is HTLV–3 antibody negative, it is still possible to have a sexual relationship without putting them at risk providing both people play safely and restrict their sexual activities to 'dry' sex which does not involve any bodily penetration or mucous membrane contact. Body to body rubbing or mutual masturbation with the use of condoms are the safest forms of sexual activity for people with HTLV–3 who have non–HTLV–3 partners.

If an infected person is not desirous or capable of sex, they shouldn't feel guilty or inadequate. Illness, emotional upset and medical treatments often reduce a person's interest in sex and their ability to have sexual responses. In the case of people with PGL, ARC or AIDS, the loss of interest in sex can be compounded by the illness being associated with sexual activity and by the fear of transmitting the virus to others or becoming exposed to opportunistic infections. Some people may find mental imagery and experimentation with erotic fantasy useful ways of overcoming sexual disinterest and strengthening sexual desire.

Home or Hospital?

If a person is seriously ill with ARC or AIDS, the question arises as to whether they ought to be cared for at home or whether it is best for them to go into a hospital.

When a person is suffering from a severe opportunistic infection such as PCP, hospitalisation is usually essential to ensure the proper monitoring and treatment of the illness. If AIDS is already so advanced that they are in a very badly weakened state – bedridden and unable to do anything for themselves – then they might also need to be cared for as an inpatient.

However, though most people with AIDS will find that a hospital stay may be necessary at some point during their illness, wherever possible it should be kept to a minimum. For as well as having the advantage of helping to cure people, hospitals also have the following disadvantages:

* They condition people to slip into the 'sick role' and to see themselves as passive 'patients'.
* They undermine a person's sense of independence and self-reliance.
* They physically isolate people from their much-needed lovers, families and friends which often causes loneliness and frustration.
* They tend to have a negative and idle atmosphere and this encourages brooding over one's own illness and the illness of others.

Thus, whenever practicable, it is advisable for a person with

AIDS to remain in or return to their own home, which usually offers a more friendly and familiar living environment with greater freedom and flexibility and more opportunity to assert one's independence. If necessary, a local authority social services department can arrange for a regular 'home help' service to supply meals and assist with shopping and home maintenance.

Patients' Rights

Whilst it is very important that a HTLV–3 infected person has a cordial and cooperative relationship with their doctor, this doesn't mean that they should uncritically accept everything the doctor says. Nearly always the doctor is right, but no one should be afraid to question a doctor's decisions or seek clarification of their advice. In particular, it is recommended that before agreeing to treatment with any of the new experimental AIDS drugs, anyone ought to seek a full explanation of the possible adverse side-effects and the possible benefits. Radiotherapy and chemotherapy, for example, which are used in the treatment of Kaposi's Sarcoma, can sometimes result in temporary skin damage, fever, hair loss, muscle aches, di-arrhoea, mouth sores, nausea, fatigue and impotence. It is, of course, true that these discomforts are well worth enduring if the treatment can reduce or eliminate the cancerous lesions. That is not, however, always the case. Certainly amongst non-AIDS cancer patients, there is a growing body of evidence that radiotherapy and chemotherapy can make some people feel worse and cause them to die sooner. In contrast, untreated cancer patients sometimes have a better quality of life and survive longer. It's therefore a good idea that you carefully weigh up the pros and cons of each therapy, and if you are unhappy you have a right to refuse or terminate treatment at any time; though this should always be done after careful consulta-tion with your doctor.

Social Security Entitlements

People with severe ARC or AIDS are sometimes no longer able to work full-time, and perhaps cannot even work at all. This can lead to serious financial problems. There are, however, a very wide range of social security benefits which are intended to help people in need and which sick people are entitled to claim. Here is a brief summary of what is available:

* *Statutory Sick Pay* is payable to most employees by their employer for the first 28 weeks of illness.
* *Sickness Benefit* is for those people not eligible for Statutory Sick Pay. It can also be claimed for up to 28 weeks.
* *Invalidity Benefit* consists of invalidity pension and an invalidity allowance which are payable indefinitely after 28 weeks of illness when a person's Statutory Sick Pay or Sickness Benefit finishes and they continue to remain incapable of working.
* *Severe Disablement Allowance* is for people who have been seriously incapacitated and unable to work for at least 28 weeks, but who can't get Sickness or Invalidity Benefit because they haven't paid enough National Insurance contributions.
* *Housing Benefit* – otherwise known as rent and rate rebates – can be claimed by both council and private tenants and by homeowners and homebuyers whose needs and financial commitments outstrip their income. It is automatically paid to people on Supplementary Benefit. Others must apply via their local council.
* *Housing Benefit Supplement* is extra help with rent and rates for people whose income is only just above the Supplementary Benefit level because, for example, they receive Invalidity Benefit. Those granted Housing Benefit Supplement are entitled to Health Benefits and may be able to claim Single Payments for special needs.
* *Supplementary Benefit* is for people who don't qualify for other benefits. It can also be paid on top of other benefits or earnings from part-time work if these are not sufficient to meet a person's needs – providing the claimant has less than £3,000 in savings. People receiving Supplementary Benefit automatically get Housing Benefit, Health Benefits and are eligible for Single Payments to meet special needs. In certain circumstances, they can also get extra weekly additions to their Supplementary Benefit for heating, laundry, diet, baths, clothing, footwear and some HP payments; plus additional allowances for blindness or near blindness, domestic assistance and attendance needs. Many of these additional weekly payments are also available to people on Housing Benefit Supplement or a low income.
* *Mobility Allowance* can be obtained by anyone who is unable, or virtually unable, to walk because of illness and who is expected to remain disabled for at least 12 months.
* *Attendance Allowance* is payable to all persons who need a lot of looking after because they have been severely sick for at

least 6 months. Prior to their eligibility for Attendance Allowance, very sick people on Supplementary Benefit, Housing Benefit Supplement or a low income can receive a weekly *Attendance Needs* payment.

★ *Invalid Care Allowance* can be awarded to people of working age who don't go to work in order to look after someone who is getting an Attendance Allowance.

★ *Health Benefits* are available to people on Supplementary Benefit, Housing Benefit Supplement and those on a low income. These benefits include: free prescriptions, glasses, and dental treatment; plus the payment of a sick person's hospital fares and those of their escort if they are unable to travel alone.

★ *Single Payments* can be made to people claiming Supplementary Benefit and Housing Benefit Supplement, but usually only if they have savings of less than £500. These one-off lump sum payments cover things like: clothing and shoes, bedding, furniture and household equipment, removal expenses, housing repairs, draught-proofing and redecoration.

If a person goes into hospital, with the exception of Statutory Sick Pay which remains unaffected, some benefits are reduced immediately, others are reduced after 8 weeks, and a few like Attendance Allowance and Invalid Care Allowance are eventually stopped altogether – though they are renewable on a person's discharge from hospital.

Owing to the highly complex nature of the social security system, frequent government changes in regulations and the variability of benefits depending on individual circumstances, it is advisable for people with ARC or AIDS to seek expert guidance from a Citizens Advice Bureau or from one of the Welfare Rights Units which have recently been set up by many local authorities.

Facing the Possibility of Death

> Death is not The End
> But the beginning
> Of a metamorphosis.
> For matter is never destroyed
> Only transformed
> And rearranged –
> Often more perfectly.

Witness how in the moment of the caterpillar's death
The beauty of the butterfly is born
And released from the prison of the cocoon
It flies free.

Given the high incidence of AIDS fatalities, people with the full-blown syndrome need to face up to the possibility, though *not* the inevitability, that they might eventually die. Not everyone can successfully fight back against AIDS. Some may try, but not pull through. There are those who, instead of resisting death, see it as a welcome release from pain and disability. Others still, having achieved many things in their life, feel at peace with themselves and are ready to die.

In her seminal work *On Death and Dying*, Dr Elizabeth Kubler-Ross suggests that people with a life-endangering illness typically experience five basic emotional reactions. These can occur separately or simultaneously, in variable order and may appear, disappear and reappear:

1) *Denial and isolation* – The person refuses to accept that the diagnosis is correct. Believing that there's been a mistake in the testing procedure or that their test results have been mixed up with someone else's, they attempt to avoid doctors and any further examinations which might reconfirm the original diagnosis. The person also withdraws from social contact and spends long periods alone.

2) *Anger* – The person feels very angry and displaces this anger onto other people in the form of resentment towards those who have good health, hatred towards those who are perceived to have caused the illness, and contempt towards the 'useless' medical profession. In addition, long suppressed anger about past personal failures and mistakes is often suddenly and explosively expressed.

3) *Bargaining* – The person seeks to delay death and extend their life to achieve a specific objective and in return promises to do something good for others. The bargain may, for example, be that if they can survive till their birthday they will donate their body to medical science or bequeath their estate to a charity.

4) *Depression* – The person experiences a 'reactive depression' at their inability to perform physical activities such as walking, cooking or dancing and their inability to fulfil their role as lover, worker or parent. They may also feel 'preparatory depression' at the prospect of their partner being left alone or their children deprived of a parent.

5) *Acceptance* – The person gradually comes to accept their illness and its possibly fatal consequences. This doesn't necessarily involve a sense of 'giving up' or 'resignation'. Acceptance can also co-exist with feelings of hopefulness about recovery and an active commitment to fighting disease.

The ability to cope with a life-threatening illness, especially in its terminal stages of development, depends a lot on a person's attitude towards death. Most people view dying as a terrible disaster. The fear, anxiety and grief it arouses often stretches deep back into a person's past and is the ultimate pained expression of a life that has been filled with cumulative losses, disappointments and unhappiness. Intensely sorrowful emotions surrounding death can also be a reflection of the regret, frustration and guilt that a person feels regarding all their mistakes, missed opportunities and uncompleted goals. Thus, coming to terms with death involves overcoming all these negative and self-denigrating feelings about one's life by learning to accept and love the self, recognising and having pride in personal achievements, healing broken relationships, and finishing one's objectives in life. These things create a sense of inner peace and strength which diminish the terror and trauma of death.

Writing about his friend's efforts in these directions, Christopher Spence recalls:

> It was very inspiring to me that, in spite of these appalling odds, Frank did fight the disease with courage and with love. He faced and felt the residual distress about his Mum's death. He worked hard at raising his self-esteem in order to combat his internalised feelings of worthlessness. He reached for people around him with powerful, cheerful loving, no matter how they treated him. He persisted in asking doctors for information (a very frightening thing for him to do). He released his feelings exhaustively whenever he could, with significant improvement in his condition (until alarmed hospital staff prescribed sufficient valium to numb out his emotions altogether). He set right his most important relationships. He was newly assertive, honest and expressive in his loving of his friends. He faced the fact that he was dying and, with characteristic precision, timed it to happen just when he had accomplished everything he needed to do first.

Coming to terms with death also involves developing new and more positive perspectives on dying: without death it would be very difficult to give life meaning or to attribute significance to personal events and achievements. Life therefore has value precisely because it is temporary and transient. On another level, we need to appreciate that to die is the destiny of all living things. Whilst some die sooner and others later, in the end death claims us all. It is the natural and inevitable conclusion to the process of living. Indeed, death is intrinsic to life itself. The decay of autumn is necessary for the birth of spring. Old leaves must fall so that new buds may grow. The caterpillar has to die before the butterfly can be born. In *Strangers Among Us*, Ruth Montgomery sums up this realisation:

> We are spirits. That bodies should be lent us while they can afford us pleasure, assist us in acquiring knowledge, or in doing good to our fellow-creatures, is a kind and benevolent act of God. When they become unfit for these purposes and afford us pain instead of pleasure, instead of an aid become an encumbrance, and answer none of the intentions for which they were given, it is equally kind and benevolent that a way is provided by which we may get rid of them. Death is that way. We ourselves, in some cases, prudently choose a partial death. A mangled, painful limb which cannot be restored we willingly cut off. He who plucks out a tooth parts with it freely, since the pain goes with it; and he who quits the whole body parts at once with all pains and possibilities of pains and diseases which it was liable to or capable of making him suffer.

Montgomery goes on to quote the following poignant epitaph:

> The Body of B. Franklin
> Printer,
> Like the Cover of an Old Book,
> Its Contents Torn Out
> And
> Stripped of its Lettering and Gilding,
> Lies Here
> Food for Worms,
> But the Work shall not be Lost
> For it Will as He Believed
> Appear Once More
> In a New and more Elegant Edition
> Revised and Corrected
> By the Author.

Shortly before he died of AIDS, William too came to a new understanding of death which enabled him to die calmly, with dignity and totally at peace with himself: 'I realised the need to accept my own impending death and physical mortality. I also realised that self-compassion meant feeling in my heart that even death was not a sign of weakness or failure. This seems to be the ultimate act of self-acceptance . . . Soon my body will be dropping away from me like a cocoon and my spirit will fly like a butterfly – beautiful and perfect. I don't claim to know exactly where it is that I am going, but my heart tells me that it is filled with light and love. An open heart is an infinitely greater blessing than death is a tragedy.' As William courageously demonstrated in the closing stages of his life, we all have choices – even in death. The process of dying doesn't have to be something that 'happens' to people as passive and powerless objects. To a significant degree, we can intervene in that process to prepare for our death so that it takes place in a way we want it and so that we avoid any disputes between family, lovers and friends about our wishes. This involves looking after practical issues such as:

★ Making a will and choosing an executor who you trust to carry out your wishes. This is particularly important for gay people whose partners will otherwise receive no legal recognition.

★ Collecting together and informing your executor of the location of key personal documents such as your will, life insurance policy, deeds to property, bank accounts, shares, tax and National Insurance statements, social security claims, HP demands, rent and rate books, mortgage papers, car or boat ownership certificates and written details of any debts owed to you or by you.

★ Deciding your funeral arrangements and specifying them in your will. Would you rather a religious or non-religious service? Do you have some favourite poetry or music which you would like to be included in the service? Is your preference for burial or cremation? Where would you like your body or ashes laid to rest?

Thinking about such issues may at first seem rather morbid and even be rather difficult. But most people find that having taken care of these details, it puts their mind at ease to feel that their death will be handled in a way which reflects their feelings and their wishes.

Coping With Caring

As much as the diagnosis of ARC or AIDS can be a traumatic experience for the person who is ill, it can also lead to great emotional strain and anguish for the person's loved ones. They suddenly have to cope with new demands and pressures posed by caring for a sick person and they have to face the possibility that someone they hold dear may eventually die.

Most of us are very unprepared for coping with serious illness and death – whether it be our own or someone else's. We often don't know how to respond to a sick person's feelings or how best to give them support. The following suggestions are therefore a useful guide to care-givers who are looking after people with ARC or AIDS:

* Encourage the person to express their feelings of loss and grief. Let them know that it is okay to be themselves and that there is no need to put up a brave front and suppress what they feel.
* Be a sympathetic ear. Listen to the person you are caring for, accept and acknowledge their feelings without judgement and respond to their expressed needs. Even if you don't like what you hear, remain understanding and avoid withdrawing from the person or rejecting their feelings.
* Share your feelings with the person, including your own sadness, anxiety and strength. This open and honest type of relationship produces closeness and bonding, thereby creating an interaction between care-giver and care-receiver which is based on partnership rather than paternalism.
* Don't 'mother' or 'baby' a person with AIDS. Treat them as a responsible adult, rather than a child or a victim. Constant 'tea and sympathy' robs the person of their self-respect and independence, inducing passivity and acceptance of the 'sick role' and reinforcing their feelings of helplessness and powerlessness.
* Be helpful and supportive of the sick person in a way which encourages their self-responsibility instead of the expectation that whenever there is a crisis you'll come running like a fire engine to the rescue.
* Reinforce the person's efforts and achievements with favourable and positive comments when they look better, stick to their exercises and diet, gain weight, increase their T helper cells and so on.
* Don't reward illness by doing everything for the person with AIDS; by insulating them from problems and bad news; or by expecting nothing from them. Acting in these ways removes their incentive to get well.
* If the sick person neglects themselves or behaves self-destructively, try not to lecture them or to force ideas upon

them. Instead, discuss the problems which are provoking this behaviour and suggest alternative ways of dealing with them.

* Do pleasurable things with the sick person apart from nursing and caring. Take a walk together in the park, go to a cricket match or visit an art gallery or cinema. This relieves the pressure of caring and shows that you value the person as a real friend, not just looking after them out of sympathy because they are sick.

Tending a person with ARC or AIDS is a tremendously draining task – both physically and emotionally. Care-givers are always in danger of over-stretching their commitment and burning themselves out by trying to do too much and being at pains to never fail. It's therefore very important that they are aware of their own vulnerability and recognise their own needs. The following tips can help make the care-giving role a little easier and a lot more effective:

* Avoid denying your own requirement of rest and relaxation and a healthy way of living. Get regular exercise and sleep, eat a nutritious diet and practise stress control and limitation. Not only will this make you feel better and enable you to nurse a person with AIDS more effectively, it will also set a positive example to the person you are caring for.

* It's dangerous to attempt to be a super-carer. Total and incessant self-sacrifice often indicates guilt and negative expectations about the person's chance of recovery. It also leaves you feeling drained, resentful and a less effective care-giver.

* Accept help when it is offered. Don't think that you are the only one who can do the job. Others can manage and the break will give you an opportunity to recover your energy.

* If help isn't spontaneously forthcoming, you shouldn't feel afraid to ask family and friends to assist. Perhaps you could also consider whether your attempt to always take charge of everything to do with the sick person is unwittingly making others feel that their help is not wanted.

* Devise strategies for coping with objectionable behaviour by the person with AIDS such as abuse and bad temper. Try, for example, leaving the room and doing a few minutes deep-breathing or meditation to calm yourself down. Then when you feel better, return to the room to show the person that you are not rejecting them.

* There is no need to hate yourself if you get angry or say the

wrong things to the person you are looking after. You are only human and sometimes you are bound to let out anger and make errors of judgement. A simple apology is adequate.

* Keep up outside social contacts and activities so that you don't become totally care-centred to the detriment of your other friends and interests. Regularly do things that give you pleasure and relief from the nursing role – buy some new clothes, have an evening out at a disco, go for a meal at your favourite restaurant or spend a day at the races.

Chapter 5

Campaigning to Defeat AIDS

> We must love one another or die.
> *W.H. Auden, 'September 1, 1939'*

Media Misrepresentation

No illness has been so inaccurately, sensationally and unsympathetically reported as AIDS. And rarely have the sufferers of any illness ever been so blatantly smeared, scapegoated and stereotyped.

For years, whilst AIDS was only killing homosexuals, the press almost totally ignored the issue. Then, suddenly, as soon as 'innocent' heterosexuals began dying from the syndrome, AIDS instantly became newsworthy. Indeed, it became Big News with a flood of shock-horror stories meriting two-inch front page headlines in the tabloid press. With all the rehearsed theatricity, prejudiced moralising and barely restrained hysteria of a gothic melodrama, papers like the *People, Sun, Star, Mirror, News of the World* and *Times* respectively thundered against 'The March Of The Gay Plague', 'Killer Sex Disease', 'Monster In Our Midst', 'The Frightening Scourge Of Our Times', 'The Gay Killer Bug' and 'Acquired Immoral Deficiency Syndrome'. To Fleet Street, AIDS was a news cocktail which embodied all the ingredients on which sensationalist journalism thrives – homosexuality, venereal disease, disfigurement, disability and death. In the words of ex-Fleet Street editor Derek Jameson, it was like a 'gift from God'. Indeed, it was, for in February and March 1985, AIDS phobia and panic was probably selling more newspapers than bingo. It became the latest weapon in Fleet Street's relentless circulation war, with the dailies feverishly competing against each other to see who could get the most sordid and morbid exclusive on what the *Sun* described as 'the scourge sweeping Britain'.

The Rev. Gregory Richards, the chaplain at Chelmsford Prison who died from AIDS in January 1985, was the subject of one of the worst of these lurid and scare-mongering Fleet Street scrambles. 'Gay Plague Kills Priest' screamed the *Sun*'s headlines. With all the drama of a Hammer horror, it went on to reveal the gruesome details: hospital staff wore 'special protective clothing' and Rev. Richard's body was stored in a 'plastic bag and deep frozen' under conditions of 'strict security' till it could be destroyed by burning for 'five times as long as normal'. Not to be outdone, the *Mirror*'s angle was that Rev. Richards was chaplain to '200 boys in his care'. The insinuation was clear, though apparently not clear enough for the *Express* whose editorial spelt it out straight: 'To allow him to work among young men passes belief. God knows how many people he may have infected.' There was, of course, not a shred of evidence that Rev. Richards had behaved improperly with any of the prison inmates, but as ever, most of Fleet Street were not going to let the facts stand in the way of a spicy and salacious story. Encapsulated within the reporting of this character-assassinating news item were the two key hallmarks of the media's misrepresentation of AIDS – the idea that the illness is a plague and contagion and that homosexuals are a threat to the health of society. The ill-founded public fear of AIDS as a rampant disease had been generated by totally unsubstantiated reports such as that which appeared in the *Express*, 'Warning of "1 Million Cases in Britain"' and by a succession of scare-mongering headlines in which the *Sun* excelled: 'It's Spreading Like Wildfire', 'Everyone Is At Risk', 'No One's Safe' and most ridiculously of all, 'Have You Got AIDS?' – as if the virus could be passed from one person to another like a common cold.

All these misconceptions about the virulence and pervasiveness of AIDS – plus a great deal of downright bigotry – have been reinforced by the way in which the disease has been dubbed 'The Gay Plague'. Quoting the Rev. Owen Leigh-Williams of St Andrew's Church, Basildon, under the headline 'AIDS Is The Wrath Of God Says Vicar', the *Sun* drew entirely fictitious parallels between AIDS and earlier contagions: 'Three hundred years ago came the Great Plague. Three hundred years before that came the Black Death.' Subsequently, the same paper was even more explicit: 'AIDS is the modern Black Death. It is spreading like a plague, threatening to strike down millions.' Similar histrionics were evident in the *Mirror*'s exaggerated revelations about 'the dreaded gay plague'. Leading in bold capitals with: '"Burn All Your Clothes" Shock At AIDS Hospital', it printed a dramatically embroidered story of how 'Panic swept through a hospital where an AIDS victim died when staff were given the chilling order "Burn your clothes and have urgent blood tests".' The staff concerned were a cleaner who had swept the AIDS patient's room and a porter who had pushed him around in a wheelchair. Neither, in fact, stood the slightest chance of infection. The consequences of this ill-informed and hyped-up reportage of the AIDS issue have been widespread public panic and prejudice. According to Richard Wells of the Royal College of Nursing, who was interviewed in the BBC2 Open Space programme broadcast on 4 November 1985:

> It makes our work tremendously difficult because every time some new headline explodes in the *Sun* or whatever, then we have numerous telephone calls from health care providers and from patients . . . and we have to spend much of our time reassuring people that what they've read is not true or only partly true, or is in fact as much a work of fiction as Alice in Wonderland.

This view was confirmed in the same programme by Professor Michael Adler who has a large AIDS caseload at the Middlesex Hospital in London. He reported:

> We've found it difficult at times to provide optimal care for our patients because people have been frightened of the risks to them by looking after patients . . . It's also, of course, had a tremendous toll on our patients themselves. I mean, it's not a very pleasant thing to know you have AIDS or have been infected with the virus. But to take on board as well as that . . . the sort of Fleet Street moralising about the gay plague is too much.

But perhaps it was the Labour MP, Chris Smith, who really hit the nail on the head: 'Whoever first decided to label it the "gay plague" had a good ear for an alliterative headline but little sense of truth or decency. When will the newspapers – with the honourable exception of the *Guardian*– wake up to the fact that gay men, along with haemophiliacs and intravenous drug users, are *victims* of this terrible disease, rather than its perpetrators?'

AIDS Discrimination

Possibly the most devastating consequence of the press hysteria over AIDS has been the large-scale discrimination which it has fostered – not just against people with AIDS, but also against those who are HTLV–3 antibody positive and against homosexuals and haemophiliacs in general on the mere suspicion that they *might* have AIDS.

The direct correlation between inflammatory press reports and increased discrimination was most clearly demonstrated in the aftermath of February and March 1985. Prior to that period, there had been relatively little newspaper coverage or public anxiety about AIDS and comparatively few cases of discrimination. However, in the wake of the deluge of sensationalist articles which appeared daily almost non-stop during these two months, a sudden and very sharp rise in prejudice occurred. Early on, there were several cases where hospital staff refused to work with AIDS patients, pathologists declined to carry out post-mortems, and undertakers rejected requests to handle the funeral arrangements of people who had died from AIDS! For a time, some ambulance drivers and fire fighters openly declared that they would not answer calls to gay premises and would not give the kiss-of-life to injured and dying people living in 'gay areas'! Two gay lovers, Mike Murphy and John Mahoney, were banned from the Cove Ivy Leaf Club in Farnborough on the pretext that they might infect the glasses! A taxi company in Streatham refused to pick up customers from the nearby Chaplin's gay club for fear that homosexuals might infect the seats! In Swansea, cleaners at the Taliesin Arts Centre threatened not to sweep out the theatre after a Gay Sweatshop performance of the anti-nuclear play *Poppies* and only reluctantly agreed after they were issued with 'rubber gloves, protective clothing and extra powerful cleansing agents'. Following the breakdown of telephone lines at the offices of London Gay Switchboard, the staff experienced great difficulties and long delays in getting them repaired because Telecom engineers were afraid they might catch AIDS by handling the receiver mouthpieces! Twenty-four year old Nicholas Lock, a chef at the Imperial Hotel in Barnstaple, was suspended from work after he took the HTLV–3 antibody test – even though his results were negative! At Hammersmith Police Station canteen, another chef, Brian Lambard, was transferred to an inferior and lower paid job when members of the CID accused him of being gay and a potential carrier of the AIDS virus! For several weeks, staff at the William Collins School in Camden stopped sending their pupils to the Oasis Baths after being told by a divisional officer of ILEA that the pool was regularly used by members of the Gay Outdoor Club and that they might have infected the water with AIDS! At another school in Hampshire, parents organised a boycott of classes when it was discovered that a nine-year old haemophiliac pupil had been exposed to the AIDS virus! After he took a HTLV–3 antibody test, Robert Hopps, a clerical assistant at the Medical Research Council – an organisation which helps fund AIDS research – was suspended from his job when other employees refused to handle telephones and letters he had touched and protested that he might 'contaminate our children'! In Southwark, a local authority personnel officer withdrew the offer of a job in an old people's home on learning that the applicant was gay and had recently attended a sexually-transmitted diseases clinic for an AIDS check-up! Despite taking a HTLV–3 antibody test and being certified negative, a gay storeman at Smith's Meters in Streatham, Barry Lawson, was sacked under the Summary Dismissal ruling which allows for instant sacking if an 'employee's performance or conduct is totally unacceptable to the company or to other employees'! British Airways has secretly introduced a ban on the employ-ment of gay cabin staff because the possibility of AIDS amongst the aircrews is seen as damaging to the proposed privatisation of BA! The Gay Teachers Group reports a 'horrifying increase in pupil abuse of gay teachers' and increased prejudice from fellow teachers including refusals to share toilets, coffee mugs and textbooks with gay staff! The British Medical Association magazine *News Review* documented cases of building contrac-tors who were unwilling to work on gay-owned premises and of works canteens where gay staff were being segregated and forced to use disposable cups! Several insurance companies, amongst them the Guardian Royal Exchange, announced that they will not give life or medical cover to people who are HTLV–3 antibody positive and some underwriters have even extended this ban to all 'suspected homosexuals'!

Even the Prison Service has been affected by the AIDS panic. Alarmed by a couple of possible AIDS cases within the prison population, warders vetoed the transfer of inmates from one prison to another, and gay prisoners have been so badly abused and humiliated – both by other inmates and by warders – that many of them have sought voluntary segregation out of fear for their lives. A letter smuggled out of Wandsworth Prison threatened to 'do away' with homosexuals unless they were isolated by the prison authorities: 'If you don't segregate them there will be trouble in the jails that you have never experienced. We will do away with them ourselves. We don't want this risk near us. Get them out of the main population now.' At Camp Hill prison on the Isle of Wight, one gay inmate, Steven Hayward, received repeated threats that he would be 'carved up' and he frequently overheard prison officers referring to gay prisoners as 'those dirty fucking queers' and 'bloody pansies spreading disease'. Despite the threats to his life, the prison governor refused Hayward's request for a transfer to another prison!

The AIDS prison scares prompted Tony Flack, president of the Association of Magisterial Officers, to warn his members: 'If a prison in your area has been in any way connected with the disease, make sure that any correspondence from that prison is separated and dealt with taking extreme care . . . any correspondence which may be in doubt could be photographed and the originals sealed in preparation for destruction. Request your cleaning staff to thoroughly disinfect areas where defendants have had prolonged contact, such as the docks, interview rooms . . . ' At a trial at St Albans Crown Court, where the defendant William McCarthy was found to have 'swellings in significant areas', two police officers escorted him into court wearing protective white hoods and masks and a prison officer refused to sit alongside McCarthy in the dock. In another court case at Horseferry Road – where the two HTLV–3 antibody positive defendants, Jimmy Murray and Gillian Hampton, appeared on shoplifting charges – police wore plastic gloves and passed documents to the magistrate with the warning: 'They have been touched by the defendants.' The police requested that the trial be held in an outdoor car park, rather than the confined space of a courtroom, to minimise the risk of infection. This request was denied by the magistrate, but she did give them permission to handcuff and hood the defendants if necessary 'so long as they are not gagged'. Because police were too scared to fingerprint Murray and Hampton, who were described as 'modern–day lepers' by their solicitor, the court was unable to hear full details of their criminal record. Though the defendants were not unwell and certainly didn't have AIDS, the magistrate asked the probation service to give them assistance in 'preparation for their next life' and suggested that a hospice be found for them.

Perhaps most alarmingly of all, gay men and haemophiliacs with HTLV–3 infection, but not with AIDS, have been refused dental and medical treatment for routine tooth extractions and hip and hernia operaions. Even uninfected gay men have been turned away from hospitals simply because they are gay and therefore automatically categorised by some doctors as suspected carriers of the virus. Dr Alex Mills of the Terrence Higgins Trust reports: 'Some people have had treatment refused. Other people have not followed the conventional course for the management of the disease. They have had delays'.

In the worst cases, this press-inspired prejudice has also resulted in a dramatic increase in attacks on gay men. Gay Switchboard noted a substantial rise in queer-bashings outside gay pubs and clubs at the height of Fleet Street's frenzied AIDS coverage. I personally experienced six of these AIDS-related attacks. The most graphic and frightening of these occurred in early March 1985. As I was walking out of Elephant and Castle tube station, I was surrounded by a gang of six youths. One of them jeered: 'Tatchell, you red poof.' Another said: 'Oh he's the one who's been in the *Sun*. We've read all about you and the gay plague.' I lightheartedly responded by suggesting 'You don't want to believe everything you read in the *Sun*.' One of the youths replied: 'The *Sun* tells the truth about you fucking queers and your filthy diseases.' Another added: 'We hate queers. All you queers should be killed before you kill us with AIDS.' With that, all six of them set on me, kicking and punching. One drew a knife and I only narrowly escaped being stabbed by running out into the road and jumping on the back of a passing bus.

Another gay man, Peter Davis, was less lucky. Warwick Crown Court heard how he was punched and killed by 18-year old Neil McDougall who was under the erroneous impression that he had caught AIDS by drinking from the same sherry bottle as Davis. After pleading guilty to manslaughter, McDougall was sentenced to a mere three months gaol in what the judge described as 'a wholly exceptional case.' Indeed, a three-month sentence *is* wholly exceptional for manslaughter!

Government Complacency

When historians document the AIDS epidemic, the Health Minister Barney Hayhoe and his predecessor Kenneth Clarke will be seen as true conservatives whose cautious instincts and personal puritanism prevented them from taking the disease seriously. Future generations will never forgive them, for had they acted quickly and decisively it would have been possible to radically limit the spread of the virus, saving many lives and forestalling much public fear and prejudice. Instead, they ended up by doing too little too late and as a result thousands of people have had to live painfully, and die, with the dreadful, but avoidable, consequences of their inaction.

In mid-1981, the American Centers for Disease Control officially reported and recognised the existence of AIDS as a specific new illness. For the first three years thereafter, the British government did nothing. Despite all the evidence from the United States where the virus was already widespread, government ministers and the Department of Health and Social Security refused to acknowledge the gravity of the public health problem posed by AIDS. In reassuring tones, a succession of officials cautioned against exaggeration and alarmism and advised doctors, AIDS organisations and journalists: 'Don't panic.'

The inadequacy of this response was glaringly obvious from 1982 when the Communicable Diseases Surveillance Centre in Britain began regularly sending reports on AIDS to the Department of Health which indicated that a serious epidemic was on the way. The government, however, still declined to act. Even a year later, when the warning signals of a major health crisis were sounding loud and clear from American doctors and US government health agencies, the British government continued to urge calm and denied that there was any need for a comprehensive programme of action.

Simultaneously with this overseas concern, during 1983 pressure steadily began to mount on the DHSS and the Health Minister from within Britain. AIDS doctors, the Haemophiliac Society, the Terrence Higgins Trust, the gay media and gay political organisations all repeatedly pressed the government to publicly fund AIDS research, counselling for people with AIDS and a health education campaign aimed at AIDS prevention. These requests were politely ignored.

In response to clear signs that haemophiliacs were being infected with the HTLV–3 virus by contaminated American-supplied Factor 8, in 1983 the Haemophilia Society called on the government to take steps to ensure prompt British self-sufficiency in blood products. Incredibly, the Department of Health still insisted: 'There is no concrete evidence that AIDS is being transmitted by American blood into Britain. No action can be taken until more information is available.'

Eventually, it took two significant deaths – one in late 1983 and the other in mid-1984 – to provoke the government to begin to act on AIDS. The two people concerned were a haemophiliac recipient of Factor 8 and a heterosexual woman. Their deaths were significant because neither were homosexual and their fate was thus clear proof that heterosexuals were at risk from AIDS too. It was almost as if AIDS had been acceptable whilst it was only claiming homosexual lives, for as soon as 'innocent' heterosexuals began to die, the Health Minister, Kenneth

Clarke, decided that something had to be done. This initial government action was not, alas, to protect homosexuals from AIDS, but primarily to safeguard the blood transfusion service and those members of the public who depend upon it. Accordingly, in 1984 gay men were officially called upon not to donate blood, and plans were drawn up to introduce the screening of all blood donations by late 1985 and to start heat-treating all Factor 8 blood products.

Despite the government's new-found sympathy for 'innocent' AIDS victims such as haemophiliacs, this sympathy did not extend as far as agreeing to finance the generalised HTLV–3 screening of the high risk haemophiliac population. Even 'innocents' were apparently not worth the expenditure of £25,000. So in June 1984 the Haemophilia Society was forced to fund the tests at its own expense. These tests eventually confirmed what the Society had long feared and what the government had long denied – namely that nearly a quarter of all haemophiliacs – about 1,000 people – had already been infected with the virus through contaminated American blood products.

It was not until the beginning of 1985 – nearly four years after the discovery of AIDS – that there was any really substantive change in the government's approach to the disease. Instead of almost total neglect, the Health Minister switched to a strategy of virus containment within the established risk groups – gay men, intravenous drug users and haemophiliacs. To this end, in early 1985 Kenneth Clarke set up the DHSS Special Advisory Committee on AIDS with the prime purpose of preventing the contamination of blood transfusions. Inevitably, most of the members appointed to the Committee had a principal interest in the protection of the blood transfusion service, rather than any understanding of or commitment to the problems faced by gay men and the urgent need for a public awareness 'safe sex' advertising campaign. As if to atone for the years of government indifference and apathy, Clarke overreacted to the new Committee's recommendations and introduced incredibly tough new guidelines for the NHS handling of blood and other bodily specimens taken from people with AIDS. These guidelines were far more stringent than those used in America and were attacked by several of the country's leading AIDS experts. As Professor Michael Adler, Dr Anthony Pinching and Dr Richard Tedder said: 'This restriction lacks scientific justification and could jeopardise clinical, diagnostic and research work.'

Pressured by the torrent of shrill and irrational AIDS coverage in the media which led to panic demands for AIDS to be made a notifiable disease, in March 1985 the Health Minister also enacted extraordinary powers to detain people with AIDS in hospital against their will; despite the recommendations of leading medical experts who felt that the voluntary system was working well and that the new compulsory powers might deter some people from coming forward for treatment. This decision made Britain the first country in the world to legislate forcible controls to deal with the disease. As one AIDS doctor noted, the detention powers were totally unnecessary and merely an attempt to appease right-wing and homophobic opinion. 'It's a political move,' he said.

During the first half of 1985, as the number of reported AIDS cases in Britain passed the 150 mark, leading hospitals caring for people with AIDS made it clear that they were becoming overwhelmed by the combination of a rapidly rising AIDS caseload and government-imposed cuts on the National Health Service. Writing in the *British Medical Journal*, Professor Hugh Dudley of St Mary's Hospital, Paddington, and Dr Geoffrey Glazer, a consultant there, claimed that they did not have the necessary equipment or staff to adequately care for AIDS patients. They urged the DHSS to 'act at once' to provide sufficient resources to ensure that the interests of people with AIDS were safeguarded and that other patients did not suffer as a result of the strain that AIDS was placing on the NHS. The government's response was not outright rejection. Instead, it was evasive and non-commital.

Following the cabinet reshuffle in mid-1985 which saw the appointment of Barney Hayhoe as Minister of Health, the government's strategy of containment was intensified with new emphasis on thwarting the 'leakage' of AIDS into the heterosexual population. Particular attention focussed on the need to prevent so-called 'bridging groups', especially bisexual men, from introducing the HTLV–3 virus from the gay community into the general population. Again, it was almost as if AIDS was tolerable providing it remained primarily amongst homosexual men, but intolerable should it spread to heterosexuals.

From a practical point of view, the fatal flaw in this government strategy of seeking to confine AIDS within the gay community was its false assumption that gay and bisexual men are only an insignificant fraction of the population who could be isolated from the rest of society. In fact, according to the standard studies of sexuality by Kinsey and by Masters and Johnson:

* 10 percent of the population are gay or predominantly gay, which gives a figure of two million adult gay men in Britain.
* 20 percent of the population are bisexual, giving a figure of four million bisexual men in Britain.
* A third of all men have a homosexual experience leading to orgasm at some point in their adult lives, which results in a figure of more than seven million men in Britain who have had, or will have, some kind of homosexual contact.

Gay sexual experiences are thus pervasive throughout much of our society, involving a very substantial minority of the population. Indeed, so far as males are concerned, they involve somewhat in excess of seven million men – a majority of whom *also* have regular heterosexual contact. This therefore means that the expectation or desire that AIDS can be contained within the gay community is a fanciful, if not downright dangerous, delusion.

The other equally delusory dimension of the new Health Minister's strategy on AIDS was his recommendation that gay men should cut down their number of sexual partners. This was little more than a piece of barely disguised moralising. Why should only gay men reduce their intimate contacts? Surely this recommendation, if valid, should apply to everyone at risk? More pertinently, however, it was ill-informed advice. The minister's call for 'fewer casual relationships' erroneously encouraged the idea that a person with a small number of partners was safe from AIDS when, in fact, even a one-off sexual experience or a totally monogamous relationship with an infected person can be sufficient to pick up the virus. The critical factor in AIDS prevention is not the *number* of sexual partners but the *way* a person has sex, and this is the point that the minister would have been better advised to emphasise. The fact that he chose instead to attack gay promiscuity was, of course, hardly surprising given his government's professed commitment to 'Victorian values'. What, however, was truly appalling about this simplistic attempt to explain and remedy AIDS was the minister's refusal to acknowledge the reason why many, though by no means all, gay men lead a promiscuous lifestyle. Whereas heterosexual relationships are legally recognised, supported through the institution of marriage and positively encouraged by media images and social expectations, homosexual relationships continue to be publicly disavowed and derided and are still subject to various judicial sanctions despite the so-called legalisation of homosexuality in 1967. With so many prejudices and penalties against gayness, a lot of homosexuals remain riven by feelings of guilt and self-devaluation which incite quick, furtive and anonymous sex and mitigate the formation of long-term gay relationships. A society which places so many obstacles in the way of homosexual love hardly has any right to turn around and condemn gay promiscuity.

In September 1985, the Health Minister finally confirmed that the screening of all blood donations for HTLV–3 antibodies would begin in October and that the HTLV–3 antibody test would become available on demand at Sexually Transmitted Disease clinics. He also announced new grants totalling £900,000 to combat AIDS. This was in addition to the £1 million which had already been allocated over previous months – mainly to the Public Health Service Laboratory for the evaluation and implementation of HTLV–3 antibody tests in the blood transfusion service. In belated response to earlier demands by hospitals bearing major AIDS caseloads, more than two-thirds of the new grants were to the Regional Health Authorities in London.

Welcome though these funds were, it soon become apparent that they were little more than emergency petty cash given the huge needs of the hospitals concerned. The North-West Thames Regional Health Authority, for example, received a grant of £275,000 to be spread amongst all the hospitals in its region. Yet just one of the health districts within the region, Bloomsbury, which includes the Middlesex Hospital, actually needed £826,000 for AIDS testing, counselling and treatment. Furthermore, what the N-W Thames Regional Health Authority gained in direct AIDS grants, it more than lost due to the government's Resource Allocation Working Party formula which is redistributing NHS finance away from the major hospitals in central London to other parts of the country. RAWP is disastrously cutting the finances of hospitals like the Middlesex precisely at a time when they desperately need more money to cope with the AIDS epidemic.

The total inadequacy of the government's funding for the fight against AIDS was evidenced by the crisis that engulfed all the major AIDS hospitals in the last quarter of 1985 – despite the Health Minister's £900,000 grant! At St Stephen's Hospital in Fulham, for instance, which was caring for 40 people with AIDS and 500 others with antibodies to the HTLV–3 virus, doctors complained that they were 'underequipped, understaffed and overworked'. As of November 1985, St Stephen's had no immunologist or facilities to conduct immune function tests on people with AIDS. Even the most elementary equipment such as cell counters to monitor the state of patients' immune systems were lacking. According to one doctor: 'Our AIDS laboratory is short-staffed. It cannot deal with the demand for HTLV–3 antibody tests. We can't even afford to buy sufficient test kits to meet the demand. If we could afford the kits, we haven't got enough staff to administer them. We urgently need a research nurse and more trained counsellors. At the moment, we only have one trained counsellor for over 500 patients.'

Even the goverment eventually realised that this alarming state of affairs was untenable and in December 1985 it announced the allocation of a further £6.3 million for the fight against AIDS – including £2.5 million for the London hospitals which are bearing the brunt of the AIDS caseload; £2.5 million for a public health education campaign; £750,000 for the screening of blood donations; £270,000 for the haemophiliac centres; and £100,000 for the training of AIDS counsellors within the NHS. Not a penny was allocated to the Terrence Higgins Trust, even though it is the country's main AIDS charity and has led the field in AIDS health education, information services and counselling support to people with AIDS. Indeed, total government grants to the Trust prior to April 1986 amounted to a meagre £35,000. Though a further £100,000 has now been given, on the basis of a minimum of 20,000 gay men who are estimated to be HTLV–3 antibody positive, this still works out at a paltry £6.75 per head. This compares very unfavourably with government funding to haemophiliac agencies which amounts to £395,000 or nearly £400 per haemophiliac infected with HTLV–3. No one be-grudges the grants to the haemophiliac population. They deserve every penny. However, the differential level of state support does reinforce the view that the government is biassed against gay men with AIDS and that in the Health Minister's eyes homosexual lives are deemed to be less valuable than heterosexual ones.

Gay Responses

In a fit of self-righteous and ignorant moralising, that once great paper, *The Times*, in an editorial on 19 February 1985, urged gay men to show 'some sense of responsibility to fellow men. This disease is capable not only of physical harm but also of dissolving the trust on which social life is built, the trust which allows us to separate and tolerate private conduct, even of an immoral or exotic kind, from the public business of society. Homosexuals thus have a double interest in impeding the disease. If they do not wish to be viewed in the public eye in the same category as biting, spitting and scratching prisoners, they will support responsible concern.'

The truth is that at least two years before either Fleet Street, or the government, woke up to the threat of AIDS, the gay and lesbian community was already taking positive action to publicise and prevent the spread of the virus – action which papers like *The Times* have consistently ignored and refused to report.

In contrast, right from the moment that AIDS was first identified in 1981, the gay press has monitored and documented the spread of the disease, progress in medical research, methods of risk reduction and the work of self-help and support organisations for people with AIDS. Unlike the mainstream media, gay publications have contributed enormously to an unprejudiced and non-hysterical understanding of the illness and its implications.

Compared with the inordinate government delays, and even the rather lethargic official response of the medical profession, gay community action on AIDS was swift and practical. In July 1982, Terrence Higgins, a 37-year old gay man, died from a Toxoplasmosis infection just two months after being diagnosed with AIDS. Angered by the inadequacy of medical monitoring and care for people with the syndrome, and distressed by the low level of knowledge about the disease within the gay community, a group of Terrence Higgins' friends decided that something had to be done. As a result the Terrence Higgins Trust was formed, with the aims of disseminating accurate information about AIDS, organising risk-reduction health education, providing help and support for people with AIDS and encouraging research into the cause and treatment of the illness. Though most of the original founders were gay, right from the outset the Trust has seen its role as helping everyone with AIDS, regardless of sexual orientation.

In spring 1983, whilst the government continued to decry the danger from AIDS, London Gay Switchboard convened the first national symposium on the disease. As a consequence of this meeting, the Trust rapidly expanded, formalising its aims and structure and incorporating the involvement of AIDS doctors and researchers for the first time. Simultaneously, as the Health Minister brushed aside all concern about the possible contamination of the blood transfusion service, the Gay Medical Association independently advised male homosexuals not to donate blood or to carry organ donor cards. This far-sighted advice, which was more than a year in advance of any official government request, probably saved hundreds more blood transfusion recipients from becoming infected with the HTLV–3 virus. To compensate for the fall-off in blood donations by gay men which followed the GMA's recommendations, Lesbian Line launched its Blood Sisters initiative to encourage lesbian blood donors; lesbians being one of the lowest AIDS-risk groups within the population.

Safeguarding the blood supply was not, however, the only issue on which the GMA was active. Concerned at the lack of government effort and the medical profession's general ignorance about AIDS, the GMA had set up an AIDS sub-committee in January 1983 to organise a two-fold campaign of AIDS education within the gay community and amongst fellow doctors. Modelled on AIDS prevention work which had been pioneered by the Gay Men's Health Crisis organisation in New York, the GMA produced 10,000 'safe sex' leaflets which were distributed in gay bars during the summer of that year. However, plans for a further print run of 100,000 were thwarted when the Metropolitan Police raided the printers and confiscated the entire stock on the grounds of obscenity. According to the then chair of the GMA, Dr Martin Hamilton-Farrell, the leaflets were 'inoffensive to the point of being dull'.

At around the same time, August 1983, to fill the void of practical information for doctors, the GMA drafted a booklet on AIDS and sought funding for its publication from the Health Education Council. Alas, the GMA's booklet proposal was treated with 'polite indifference', as was its suggestion for a government-funded AIDS education campaign targeted at the gay community. When the GMA's proposals were referred to the DHSS, they were informed that a special booklet on AIDS was 'not necessary'. Subsequently, however, the DHSS has belatedly recognised this need and has issued a total of three booklets and advice notes to doctors! The GMA's recommendations for an AIDS awareness advertising campaign were also dismissed by the DHSS as 'premature'. Nearly three years later, the government eventually launched its own 'Don't Aid AIDS' education campaign!

From 1983, as the Health Minister dithered indecisively, the Terrence Higgins Trust grew from strength to strength and became the *only* organisation in the country with a thought-out and comprehensive strategy for tackling AIDS. It is no over-estimation to say that the officers of the Trust were far better informed and certainly more far-sighted than the government ministers and DHSS officials who were entrusted with the public health. Astonishingly, long before the government or the medical profession ever took a similar initiative, it was under the Trust's auspices that two national conferences on AIDS were convened in 1984 and 1985, bringing together AIDS doctors and researchers, haemophiliac agencies, counselling bodies and gay community organisations.

Though it has only two full-time paid workers, through its 300 volunteers the Trust organises a wide variety of activities – self-help and mutual support groups for people with AIDS and those who are HTLV-3 antibody positive; a 'buddy' system to provide companionship and home help for people with AIDS; a telephone 'helpline' for information and advice on AIDS; legal support for people with AIDS who face discrimination; and an AIDS prevention campaign promoting 'safe sex' via press advertisements, posters and leaflets – over 150,000 of which have been distributed nationwide. To finance all these activities, the Trust is almost entirely dependent on voluntary donations and fund-raising with the gay and lesbian communities. Indeed, in the last three years prior to April 1986, the homosexual community raised nearly three times as much money for the fight against AIDS as the government made available to the Trust in grants.

Of all its work, probably the most effective has been the Trust's health education campaign which has sought to encourage gay men to avoid playing dangerously. As a result, the incidence of sexually transmitted diseases amongst homosexuals has been steadily falling for the last two years in contrast to the heterosexual population in which these continued to rise. Indeed, in 1985 alone the incidence of gonorrhea amongst gay men dropped by over a third! The increase in new AIDS cases also appears to be slowing down and levelling out at around 25 per month rather than rapidly rising in an uncontrolled geometric expansion as many were predicting. These factors provide concrete evidence that the Trust's 'safe sex' advertising campaign *is* working and that gay men *are* acting responsibly by switching to less risky forms of sex.

The irony of all this is that while so much of the media has eagerly heaped the blame for AIDS onto gay men and let a complacent government completely off the hook, and while so many self-appointed moral pundits have raged against 'irresponsible' homosexual behaviour, it has actually been gay people themselves who have shown the greatest measure of responsibility, concern and practical effort to defeat AIDS. On this issue, at least, the gay and lesbian communities have asserted a moral leadership which has been singularly lacking from other quarters in society. Even the church, which is so often keen to assume moral authority, has shown an abject lack of public compassion for people with AIDS and has remained sickeningly silent regarding the cruel discrimination they have endured. How paradoxical it is that homosexuals, the subjects of such fierce clerical condemnation, should turn out to be more fitting custodians of the Christian spirit of the 'Good Samaritan' and the ideal that we are each 'Our Brother's Keeper'.

A Programme of Action Against AIDS

Given that almost everyone is now finally agreed on the massive scale of the health problem posed by AIDS, it is extraordinary that the government is *still* doing so little, more than five years after the disease was first recognised. Incredibly, despite nearly 400 cases of AIDS and up to 50,000 people infected with the virus, the Health Minister has no coherent, comprehensive and coordinated strategy either for the prevention of AIDS, the treatment of people infected with HTLV–3, or the development of a vaccine and cure for the syndrome. So far, the government has allocated a pathetic £8.6 million to combat this 'killer disease', which compares very unfavourably with President Reagan's $193 million AIDS budget for 1986 and is one of the smallest amounts spent on fighting AIDS by any comparable Western country. This penny-pinching shortsightedness may save a few pounds now, but it will end up costing the country many more millions in the future – not to mention the immense cost in terms of human suffering. It therefore makes sense, especially from the government's own monetarist perspectives, for the Health Minister to spend more on fighting AIDS today in order to save even greater expenditure in years to come. To this end, the government urgently needs to formulate and fund a concerted AIDS strategy based on the following six areas of action:

Increased finance for AIDS research

It is difficult to believe that the government is serious about defeating AIDS when one considers that the sum total of its expenditure on research into finding a vaccine or cure is a derisory £400,000. As a result, key AIDS research establishments are dependent on gay people organising fund-raising benefits and shaking collection tins in gay clubs to finance their vital work. This is the case at the Jefferiss Research Wing at St Mary's Hospital, Paddington, where they are engaged in crucial experiments on virus identification, isolation, testing and treatment; and also at King's College Hospital in Camberwell where Dr Tom McManus is doing research into gay men's sexual behaviour and lifestyle which may throw some light on why only a small proportion of people with HTLV–3 infection later go on to develop AIDS. Both establishments are being hampered in their efforts by a chronic lack of government funding.

To remedy this woeful and irresponsible neglect of AIDS research, at the very least the government needs to make available an annual budget totalling £10 million. That sounds a lot, but by comparison to what is needed and what other countries are spending, it is in fact quite a modest sum.

Direct grants to AIDS hospitals

AIDS testing, counselling and treatment is now placing a very major strain on the resources of key hospitals such as the Middlesex, St Mary's and St Stephen's. At the Middlesex Hospital, for example, because of a shortage of secretarial staff, some of the country's top AIDS doctors are forced to waste precious hours doing their own typing and filing when their efforts would be far more profitably spent on doing research and clinical work with their patients. Worse still, their AIDS laboratory is a temporary portakabin stuck on the roof of the STD clinic and it is so underequipped and understaffed that the doctors there are unable to fulfil the safety guidelines demanded by the Advisory Committee on Dangerous Pathogens. According to one doctor: 'If we obeyed the guidelines to the letter, we could not operate our laboratory and service our AIDS patients. The laboratory urgently needs upgrading.'

The National Union of Public Employees, which represents health workers in the NHS, has estimated that it costs £20,000 to care for each person with AIDS and that as many as 3,000 people may be diagnosed with the syndrome over the next two years. On these calculations, the NHS will need to spend £60 million on AIDS patient care by the beginning of 1989.

In these circumstances, the government's current policy of intermittent one–off grants, such as those disbursed to the

112

Thames Regional Health Authorities in late 1985, is simply not adequate. To cope with the acute and growing financial problems which AIDS is creating, a direct grant fund of £10 million a year ought to be set aide to assist those hospitals whose resources are being severly stretched by the combination of a rapidly growing AIDS caseload, government-imposed cuts in the NHS and the fiscally crippling effects of the ongoing redistribution of money away from the big NHS hospitals in inner London. Such a fund could also be used to overcome the existing London bias of AIDS treatment by financing the establishment of regional AIDS specialist hospitals in cities such as Cardiff, Manchester and Edinburgh.

AIDS awareness advertising

A programme of generalised public health education about AIDS could do a lot to calm popular hysteria regarding the illness, lessen the unwarranted prejudice against people who have been in contact with the HTLV-3 virus, and contribute to AIDS prevention by advising people on practical ways of reducing their risk of infection such as the use of condoms during sex. The government's allocation of a meagre £2.5 million for its 'Don't Aid AIDS' advertising campaign is a mere drop in the ocean. It means that there will not be sufficient money to run the adverts on television and radio and that the press adverts will only be repeated twice during the whole year. Doing the campaign on the cheap has also meant that the adverts have been badly designed, and because they are dull and boring they are unlikely to be effective in getting the message across, especially to the sexually active 'at risk' teenage population. To be really effective, the government needs to invest somewhere in the region of £10 million for an AIDS awareness campaign involving a continuous series of eye-catching and punchy newspaper, television and radio advertisements; plus leaflets, posters, street billboards and an education programme within schools and universities.

Similar campaigns in major American cities have proven highly successful in helping to reassure an anxious public and get across the messages: 'Play Safely' and 'Don't Share Needles'. In Los Angeles, for example, the government-funded AIDS Project has pioneered a highly imaginative 'safe sex' advertising campaign fronted by 'Mother' – a sweet, diminuitive, middle-aged housewife – portrayed by the actress Zelda Rubinstein who starred in the film *Poltergeist*. She is everyone's picture of an ideal mum and in a series of press and broadcasting adverts she lovingly urges her tall, musclebound gay sons to 'Play Safely', 'Keep It Clean' and 'Don't Forget Your Rubbers'. The same messages are repeated in pamphlets, posters and even giant street billboards which depict a gay American family – Mother surrounded by six gay sons – captioned with the slogan: 'Play Safely. LA CARES . . . Like a Mother'. To popularise 'safe sex', the AIDS Project has also printed an eight-page giveaway pamphlet, *Mother's Handy Sex Guide*, which includes three erotic stories designed to show that far from being dull, 'Playing Safely' can be very sexually exciting.

So has the AIDS Project campaign worked? Certainly, by comparison to many other US cities and to Britain there seems to be much less public panic in Los Angeles and a generally better informed public perception of AIDS. With regard to AIDS prevention, one of the Project's senior workers, John Mortimer, sums up the advertising campaign as having 'succeeded in creating an atmosphere in which it is acceptable to talk about "Playing Safely"; where people are not going to be put down for wanting to reduce their risk of AIDS.' He is also convinced that by persuading more and more people to give up dangerous sexual practices, 'safe sex' advertising has already started to slow down the spread of the virus. It is certainly evident amongst gay men in Los Angeles that by comparison to a few years ago there is much less cruising and a lot more socialising with friends. Increasingly, gay men are dating before sex and getting into deeper, long-term love affairs. Greater value is being placed on caring, supportive friendships. Responsibility is becoming the catchword in personal relationships and, in echoes of the 1950s, romance is back in fashion.

There has been no exhaustive survey of the precise effect of Mother's 'Play Safely' campaign on gay men's sexual habits in Los Angeles. However, a poll taken in 1985 by the AIDS Foundation in San Francisco revealed that following a similar AIDS awareness advertising campaign 81 percent of gay men in the city had adopted 'safe sex' practices. These figures are borne out by statistics from San Francisco's main STD clinic which show that the incidence of rectal gonnorrhea has dropped by 86 percent in recent years. The lessons from both Los Angeles and San Francisco seem clear: in the absence of an AIDS vaccine or cure, a well-funded government-sponsored health education campaign can play a crucial role in restricting the spread of the virus, saving many lives and much money in the long run. It's a positive lesson which the British government's miserly 'Don't

Aid AIDS' campaign has only half-heartedly acknowledged.

Public funding for AIDS organisations

To fill the void created by government inaction against AIDS, not only was the Terrence Higgins Trust established, but in its wake a growing number of local AIDS organisations have also been set up such as Reading AIDS Inquiry Line, Scottish AIDS Monitor, Manchester AIDS Line, OxAIDS, Plymouth AIDS Support Group, Merseyside AIDS Helpline and so on. All these organisations, doing things that are really a government or local authority social services responsibility, operate primarily on voluntary effort and donations. Despite generous support from the gay and lesbian communities, they still suffer from chronic under-funding and are therefore unable to offer the full range of services that they would wish and that an AIDS-anxious public is demanding.

In the case of the Terrence Higgins Trust, which is the country's premier AIDS charity, the organisation's entire operation is run from two tiny offices, separated by a corridor, in a former warehouse off Gray's Inn Road. The Trust has only two full-time paid staff, no interview or counselling rooms and only one small space downstairs which acts as meeting place for its AIDS support groups. To overcome these limitations, the government urgently needs to allocate an annual grant of £1 million to the Trust for the purposes of enabling it to:

* Move into larger premises with adequate space for administrative offices, the telephone helpline service, an AIDS monitoring and information library, and interview, counselling and meeting rooms.
* Open a 'drop in' centre for off-the-street inquiries from the public and a meeting place where people who have AIDS or are HTLV-3 antibody positive can socialise in a friendly and relaxed environment.
* Finance administrative expenses and purchase desperately needed office equipment such as an electronic stencil cutter and a high-speed duplicator.
* Expand the telephone helpline to a 15 hours a day, seven days a week nationwide freephone service.
* Employ 12 new staff including one director, one press and publicity officer, one 'buddy' programme and support group coordinator, three professional counsellors and six trained telephone helpline receptionists.

* Organise specialist AIDS risk-reduction advertising campaigns targeted at high-risk groups such as gay men and
  intravenous drug users.

Additionally, a further yearly government grant of £250,000
ought to be spread amongst the other local AIDS organisations
in the out-of-London regions to enhance their ability to service
their own populations and to supplement the often negligible or
non-existent local authority funding which is now being made
more and more difficult by government-imposed cuts in the rate
support grant and the strictures of rate-capping.

Guarantee of confidentiality and repeal detention powers

Soon after the government introduced its draconian powers to
detain people with AIDS in hospital against their will, in March
1985, Roger, a 29-year old AIDS patient in Manchester, was
forcibly confined in Monsall Hospital. This confinement was
largely due to panic by the public authorities and the failure of
doctors to adequately explain to Roger that given his state of
ill-health he may have placed himself and others at risk by
voluntarily discharging himself. The use of these powers thus
could have been avoided by a more sympathetic and sensitive
relationship with the patient.

The detention powers are, however, not only unnecessary,
they are also downright harmful to the task of controlling the
spread of AIDS. So, too, is the mounting pressure for doctors to
be legally compelled to breach patient confidentiality by
informing the spouses of people with HTLV–3 infection
without the person's knowledge and regardless of their wishes.
Both these practices risk discouraging people from coming
forward for testing and treatment, either out of fear that they
may be held in hospital against their will or that others will be
informed about their condition without their agreement. For
this reason, to ensure total confidence in AIDS screening and
treatment and maximum public cooperation in controlling
AIDS, the government must act at the earliest opportunity to
repeal the detention powers and reaffirm its commitment to
stand by the principle of undiminished patient confidentiality.

A ban on AIDS discrimination

People with AIDS – and those with PGL, ARC and HTLV–3
antibody positive status – have to cope with a double burden.
Not only must they face the trauma of a life-threatening illness,

but increasingly this hardship is being compounded by the experience of prejudice, ostracism and discrimination – the stressful effects of which can often exacerbate their illness. It is therefore imperative that both central and local government promptly legislate to ban all discrimination in the fields of employment, housing, education and the provision of public and private services – with the sole exception of certain limited categories of services such as blood, organ and sperm donation.

Already, some US cities, notably Los Angeles and its neighbourhood city of West Hollywood, have enacted similar anti-AIDS discrimination ordinaces. West Hollywood, for example, has prohibited discrimination against 'persons suffering from AIDS and AIDS-related conditions, carriers of the virus that causes AIDS, and persons regarded by others as having AIDS'. The ban on discrimination covers the fields of 'employment, housing, business establishments, health care services, city facilities and services and other public services and accommodations'. Aggrieved persons are empowered to sue for up to $10,000 in damages.

In Britain, government ministers have it within their power to save thousands of lives and hundreds of millions of pounds by acting *now* to implement this coherent, comprehensive and coordinated strategy to conquer AIDS. Blinded, however, by their own narrow personal prejudices and a dogmatic adherence to mean-fisted public expenditure policies, it seems that ministers are unable, or reluctant, to act with foresight and vigour. The question is: how many more people will have to die before the government is prepared to wholeheartedly tackle AIDS by putting the necessary resources into defeating this dreadful disease and the equally dreadful panic and prejudice it has generated?

> Look to this day, it is life.
> For yesterday is already a dream
> and tomorrow is only a vision.
> But today, if well lived, makes every
> yesterday a dream of happiness,
> and every tomorrow a vision of hope.
> *Sanskrit Proverb*

The activities listed in these appendixes are equally applicable to people who are HTLV–3 antibody positive as well as those with PGL, ARC, and the full AIDS syndrome. They require perseverance. Don't expect instant results. If done regularly, however, these activities can help enhance the quality of your life, improve your health, and increase your chances of survival.

You cannot hope to do all the activities every day. Concentrate on doing the most important ones – *affirmation meditation, mental imagery* and the *work-out*. Do the others as the opportunity or need arises. If, for example, you find your energy flagging by mid-afternoon, do some Qi Gong to relax and refresh. And if you've had a hard day and feel stressed, in the early evening try the relaxation exercises or meditation to unwind.

Draw up a day planner

Morning	– Affirmation Meditation (5 minutes)
	– Mental Imagery (10 minutes)
	– Work-Out (10–15 minutes)
	– Inspirational Music (5 minutes)
Lunch Break	– Mental Imagery (10 minutes)
Afternoon Tea Break	– Qi Gong (10 minutes)
Early Evening	– Relaxation Exercises or Relaxation Meditation (15 minutes)
Bed Time	– Mental Imagery (10 minutes)
	– Body Massage or Relaxation Exercises or Relaxation Meditation or Relaxing Music (15 minutes)

NB: The duration and number of repetitions for the various activities listed in these appendixes are minimum suggestions. You can, however, adapt them to your own needs and desires. If, for example, you find affirmation meditation particularly helpful, you might want to lengthen it to 10 minutes per session or repeat it in the evening before bed.

Appendix 2
Affirmation Meditation

In affirmative meditation, by reciting an affirmation which embodies your will to live and thinking about positive future goals, you gather mental strength and create feelings of self-confidence which assist physical recovery.

Instructions

1) Meditate in a pleasing environment which is quiet and darkened.
2) Sit cross-legged on the floor with your eyes closed.
3) Clench and then slowly relax your muscles – feel them growing loose and limp.
4) Breathe deeply in and out through your nose for 2 minutes. As you inhale, concentrate on the sound of your own breath. As you exhale, think of the word 'relax'.
5) Slowly, with great concentration, mentally recite your affirmation and carefully contemplate its meaning. If you wish, recite more than one affirmation or vary the affirmations each day.
6) Spend a minute thinking about the positive goals that you want to achieve in the day ahead and in the coming months.
7) Conclude with 30 seconds of deep breathing.
8) Repeat this meditation every morning when you wake up.

Choose from the following affirmations, or write your own, and learn them off by heart:

A Positive Attitude

I have a positive attitude – the determination to survive.
I believe in myself and my ability to fight this disease.
I possess the mental and physical strength to conquer adversity.
I am not a 'victim' and I do not accept the 'sick role'.
I know it is still possible to live an enjoyable and worthwhile life.
I can and will retain mastery and control over my future.
Today I will take care of myself and the people I love.
Today I will eat a nutritious diet.
Today I will get plenty of sleep and lots of exercise.
Today I will avoid stress and seek relaxation.
Today I will do things which bring me – and others – happiness.
I am, I can, I will.

Take Time

Today I shall . . .
Take time to THINK – It is the origin of wisdom and power.
Take time to WORK – It is the price of success.
Take time to PLAY – It is the secret of vitality and relaxation.
Take time to BE FRIENDLY – it is the door to happiness.
Take time to GIVE – It is the source of mutual joy.
Take time to LOVE and BE LOVED – It is the greatest healer.
Take time to HOPE – It is the key to survival.
Take time to CARE – It is the foundation of a future worth living for.

I Have the Will

I have the will to live.
Not merely to linger and survive.
But to live life to the full –
To be valuable and productive
As I fight and stay alive.

To Try

No future is too hopeless
No struggle is too arduous
No goal is too remote
No obstacle is too great.
In short, there is nothing
Too overwhelming,
Or too overawing,
To stop me from trying.

I Shall

I shall repeatedly challenge and never give in
I shall remain defiant and refuse to let go
I shall believe in myself and tell death 'No!'
For I am full of optimism and sure I can win.

Relaxation Meditation

Relaxation meditation is a way of liberating the mind from all distracting and disturbing thoughts and emotions to achieve a sense of inner mental calm and happiness. This assists the process of emotionally coping with a life-threatening illness and by reducing stress it boosts the body's natural resistance to disease.

Method

Follow instructions 1–4 in Affirmation Meditation: choose a quiet and darkened room. Sit in a comfortable chair or cross-legged on the floor with your eyes closed, shoulders relaxed and hands resting on your legs. Do a couple of minutes of deep-breathing and muscle-relaxing exercises to get yourself feeling mentally and physically at ease.

Each of the following relaxation meditation exercises should be continued for 5–10 minutes:

Relaxation meditation using fantasy

Visualise yourself in paradise. Picture it as the most beautiful and tranquil place on earth. Savour its every sensation. Perhaps it is a beach – imagine the sun's rays warming your body, the soft white sand caressing your skin, and the cool water lapping over your limbs. Or maybe your paradise is an alpine meadow – feel yourself inhaling the bracing mountain air, drinking the fresh spring water, and scenting the aroma of a field filled with exquisite wild flowers.

A slight variation on this meditation is free-association fantasy. Instead of the mind being consciously directed to the creation of a specific fantasy paradise, with the aid of music it is encouraged to roam free and conjure up its own mental fantasies from deep inside the unconscious. For this purpose, electronic synthesiser music is ideal: Jean Michel Jarre's *Oxygen*, Kraftwerk's *Trans-Europe Express*, Mike Oldfield's *Tubular Bells*, David Bowie's *Heroes* and the musical scores from films such as *2001*, *A Clockwork Orange*, *Star Wars* and *Close Encounters of the Third Kind*.

Relaxation meditation using repetitive sounds, words or visual images

With intense concentration, mentally or verbally repeat over and over again the same sound or word. It could be a meaningless sound like 'Ummm' or 'Ahhh'. Or it could be a goal-suggestive word like 'relax' or 'calm'. A visual variant on this technique involves picturing the mind as a black velvet expanse or an endless still lake of black ink.

Relaxation meditation using repetitive mental exercises

- Sit cross-legged on the floor with your eyes closed.
- Imagine that a small heavy ball, a little bigger than a tennis ball, is resting on the palms of your hands.
- Slowly, as you inhale, raise the ball up to your chest.
- Then roll your hands and arms over the ball so that it is pressing up heavily on the palms.
- Slowly, as you exhale, lower your hands and press the ball downwards to its original position.
- Roll your hands and arms under the ball and repeat 30 times.
- After you have got used to this technique, imagine that the ball is inside your abdomen. Move it up and down in synchronisation with your breathing, but without the aid of your hands.

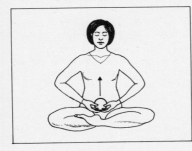

INHALE

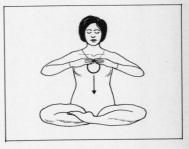

EXHALE

With so many different meditative methods to choose from, it is advisable to experiment to determine which one suits you best.

Mental Imagery

Mental imagery is a method of strengthening your 'will to live' and affirming your belief that you *can* survive. Because it gives a new-found sense of participation and control over the process of recovery, mental imagery can boost self-esteem and reduce feelings of stress, fear and helplessness – thereby improving the functioning of the immune system.

Technique

1) Choose a pleasant room where it is dark and quiet.
2) Sit cross-legged on the floor and close your eyes.
3) Tense your muscles, then very slowly 'let go' and feel yourself becoming relaxed.
4) Breathe deeply through your nose for 2 minutes. Concentrate on the sound of your own breath as you breathe in, and mentally repeat the word 'relax' as you breathe out.
5) In *realistic* cell-like form visualise your body fighting back against AIDS:
   * Mentally picture the AIDS viruses as being small in size and number – weak, isolated and vulnerable.
   * If you have an opportunistic infection such as pneumonia, or a cancer such as Kaposi's Sarcoma, imagine its cells likewise feeble and few.
   * Then picture your immune system as a vast mass of invincible defender cells:
     – Imagine your T helper cells rapidly multiplying, growing large and strong, and switching on your immune system.
     – Imagine your scavenger and killer cells aggressive and immensely powerful.
     – Imagine your B cells producing millions of potent antibodies.
   * Next, picture the masses of scavenger, killer and B cells overwhelming and destroying the AIDS viruses/opportunistic infections /cancers.
   * Simultaneously, picture any medical treatment you are having as coming into your body to assist the efforts of your defender cells by swamping and poisoning the AIDS viruses/opportunistic infections/cancers.
   * When *all* the AIDS viruses/opportunistic infections/cancers have been destroyed, picture them as debris being carried away in your bloodstream, filtered out by your kidneys and liver, and excreted from your body in urine and faeces.
   * And finally, picture your body purified, strong and healthy. Imagine yourself with your goals in life accomplished. See yourself happy, surrounded by the people you love.

NB: If you have difficulty in picturing the above effects, try feeling them instead. Imagine, for example, what it would feel like to be fit and full of energy.

6) Now visualise your body fighting back against AIDS in *symbolic* fantasy form:

* You could, for example, picture the AIDS viruses/opportunistic infections/cancers as a small group of languid squids and your defender cells as a huge shoal of sharks. Imagine the sharks ferociously devouring *all* the squids and not letting a single one escape. Then picture the sharks swimming away and the sea becoming totally tranquil and crystal clear to reveal an exotic wonderland of filagree corals and tiny multicoloured fish shimmering in the warm aquamarine waters.

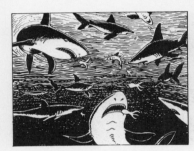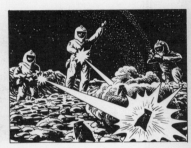

* An alternative symbolism could be based on warfare – 'AIDS Wars' – in which the defender cells are represented by huge cosmic armies of white galactic knights who attack with laser weapons, sizzling and vapourising *all* the little legless space creatures which represent the AIDS viruses/opportunistic infections/cancers. After the 'AIDS Wars' are over, imagine the quiet deserted battleground blooming into life – a lush 'Garden of Eden' filled with exquisite flowers and bathed in the breathtaking beauty of an interstellar sunset.

  NB: These symbolic images are only suggestions. Choose whatever imagery you feel happiest with.

* Finally, picture your health recovered – your body powerful, your goals in life achieved, and your personal relationships fulfilling and joyful.

7) Conclude the mental imagery with a minute's deep breathing.

8) Repeat 3 times a day for 10 minutes using *either* realistic *or* symbolic imagery – whichever suits you best.

9) Once a week, do a drawing of your mental imagery and display it prominently in your home as a visual reminder of your commitment to overcoming AIDS.

Most people find mental imagery quite difficult to begin with, but it gets easier with practice and after a couple of weeks it should start having a noticeable effect.

Exercise creates suppleness, stamina and strength. It can also help relieve tension, improve circulation and oxygenate the blood, and enhance the body's natural defences against infection.

Instructions

* Exercise every morning for 10–15 minutes before breakfast.
* Wear a loose-fitting T-shirt and shorts.
* Exercise in a bright, spacious room with the windows wide open to allow in plenty of fresh air.
* Put on some lively disco music to get yourself in an energising mood.
* Precede the exercises with 2 minutes of deep breathing.
* Then progress to the 4 warm-ups, followed by the 4 work-outs.
* Do the Day 1 exercises on Mondays, Wednesdays and Fridays, and the Day 2 exercises on Tuesdays, Thursdays and Saturdays. Rest on Sundays.

Exercise tips

* Keep breathing steadily – exhaling as you exert and inhaling between exertions.
* Push yourself to the limit, but never overstrain or exercise to the point of exhaustion. A healthy work-out should leave you feeling pleasantly tired – not shattered.
* If you are very unfit or already ill, only do a couple of the less strenuous warm-ups to start with. Then *gradually* increase the numbers and progress to the more difficult work-out exercises as you gather strength.
* Some of the exercises are quite hard to do. Don't be deterred if, at first, you can't do them properly or can only do a couple of repetitions. Think of the exercises as a target to aim for. With perseverance, in six weeks you should be able to do them all. You'll also look better and feel better too!

DEEP BREATHING EXERCISES

1) Stand feet together and arms by your side.
2) Slowly breathe in through your nostrils – lifting and expanding your chest – to fill your lungs with as much air as possible.
3) Hold your breath briefly.
4) Then breathe out slowly and firmly through your mouth till every last bit of air is expelled from your lungs and your chest is deflated and compressed.
5) Repeat 10 times.

Alternating deep breathing

A) As above, but cover the left nostril with the left hand.
B) Breathe in through the right nostril and hold briefly.
C) Remove the left hand and place the right hand over the right nostril.
D) Breathe out through the left nostril.
E) Then reverse – keep the right nostril covered with the right hand.
F) Breathe in through the left nostril and hold briefly.
G) Remove the right hand and place the left hand over the left nostril.
H) Breathe out through the right nostril.
I) Repeat 10 times.

Day 1 – Warm-Ups

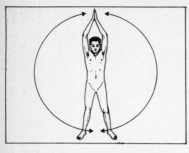

1) HAND CLAPS (OVERHEAD AND BEND DOWN). Stand with feet apart. Keeping arms straight at all times, clap palms of hands firmly together above head. Then simultaneously lower arms sideways and bend downwards to clap palms of hands together again just above ground. Repeat 10–30x.

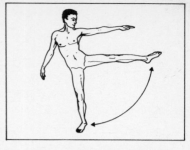

2) LEG RAISERS (SIDEWAYS). Stand with feet together. Hold body vertical and, keeping both legs straight, slowly lift left leg sideways to horizontal position. Point toes and hold. Lower leg. Repeat 5–30x. Then switch to right leg.

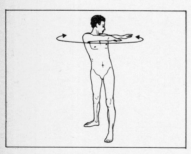

3) BODY TWISTS. Stand with feet apart. Keeping arms parallel with ground and feet stationary, swing both arms leftwards as far back as possible. Press 3x hard to left. Then swing arms around and press 3x hard to right. Repeat 5–30x.

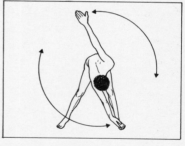

4) TOE TOUCHES. Stand with feet apart. Bend down and simultaneously touch left toe with right hand whilst raising left arm behind back. Then lower left hand to touch right toe whilst raising right arm behind back. Repeat 10–30x.

Day 1 – Work-Out

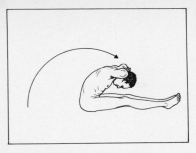

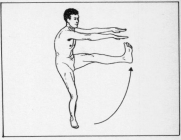

1) SIT-UPS. Lie on back with hands clasped behind neck. Keeping back straight, sit up and bend forward to touch knees with forehead (ensuring that knees remain flat on ground and elbows point sideways). Lie down. Repeat 10–40x.

2) HIGH KICKS. Stand with feet together and arms outstretched in front. Keeping both legs straight, kick left leg forwards to touch finger-tips of right hand. Lower leg to standing position. Then kick right leg to touch left finger-tips. Repeat fast 5–30x.

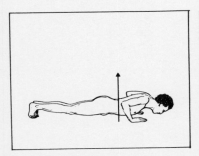

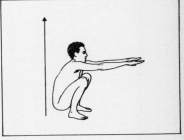

3) PUSH-UPS. Facing downwards, balance on toes and palms and put all weight on outstretched arms. Keeping body straight, compress arms and lower body to almost touch ground. Then use arm muscles to push body upwards till arms are fully extended. Repeat 5–30x.

4) SQUATS. Stand with feet apart and arms held forward. Keeping back straight and feet flat on ground, squat down till buttocks touch heels. Then, using leg muscles, push upwards and return to standing position. Repeat 5–30x.

Day 2 – Warm-Ups

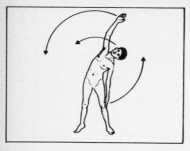

1) SIDE STRETCHES. Stand with feet apart. Without leaning forward, bend left arm sideways over head. Press hard 3x in a rightwards direction whilst simultaneously 3x forcing right arm downwards along calf of right leg. Then switch to right arm. Repeat 5–30x.

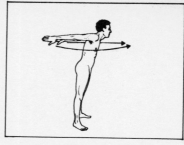

2) HAND CLAPS (BACK AND FRONT). Stand with feet apart. Keeping arms straight and completely horizontal, clap palms of hand firmly together behind back. Then clap them together again in front. Repeat with speed 5–30x.

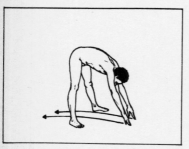

3) GROUND TOUCHES. Stand with feet wide apart. Bend over. Keeping legs straight and both arms close together, stretch forwards to touch ground. Then swing arms between legs and stretch backwards to touch ground. Repeat in swinging motion with speed 10–40x.

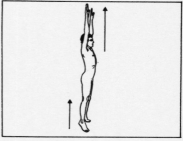

4) SKY REACHES. Stand with feet apart on tiptoes. Hold both arms vertically above head. Stretch whole body upwards as if trying to reach sky till muscle strain is felt all over. Hold 10 seconds, then lower feet and arms. Repeat 5–30x.

Day 2 – Work-Out

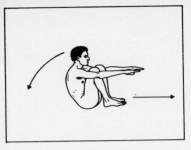

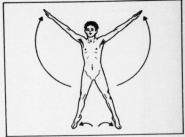

1) BODY TUCKS. Sit balanced on buttocks with arms outstretched in front and knees tucked up into chest. Simultaneously extend legs forwards till fully straight and lie backwards – but without letting feet or shoulders touch ground. Resume original body tuck position. Repeat 5–30x.

2) LEG SPRINGS. Stand with feet together and arms by side. Simultaneously spring both legs apart and lift arms sideways above head. Then spring legs together again and lower arms by side. Repeat in rapid bouncing movements 10–40x.

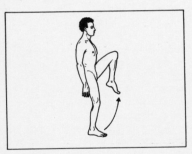

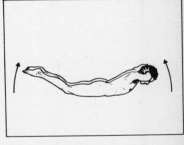

3) KNEE LIFTS. Stand with feet together and arms by side. Keeping back straight and pointing toes downward, raise left knee to touch left shoulder. Then lower. Do likewise with right knee. Repeat with speed 5–30x.

4) BACK ARCHES. Lie on the ground face downwards with toes pointed and hands clasped behind neck. Keeping elbows level with shoulders, simultaneously lift legs and top half of body off ground as high as possible so that back arches and body balances on hips. Lower to ground. Repeat 5–30x.

Relaxation Exercises

Relaxation exercises can help alleviate muscle tension and ensure a deeper, more relaxed sleep; thus strengthening the body's ability to fight off infection.

Technique

1) Choose a warm, quiet and dark room.
2) Loosen any constricting clothes.
3) Ensure adequate ventilation – without draughts.
4) Stand with your feet apart.
5) Start, eyes closed, with 3 minutes of deep breathing exercises – inhaling and exhaling through your nose without holding your breath. Each time you breathe out, mentally say the word 'relax' and imagine your body growing limp and heavy.
6) Then, one by one, shake your hands, feet, arms and legs till they feel loose like a trouser-leg.
7) Now you are ready to commence the relaxation exercises 1–14.
8) Do all exercises in slow, rhythmic motions.
9) Repeat each exercise as many times as necessary till all tension disappears and you feel relaxed.
10) Throughout each exercise, keep your eyes closed and block out all other thoughts by concentrating on the movements of the exercise in question.
11) Conclude by lying on the bed/floor and closing your eyes –
   * Working from the head to the toes, mentally check that every part of your body is relaxed.
   * Wherever there is residual tension, clench the tense area and then relax. Alternatively, imagine the taut muscle as a clenched fist and visualise it gradually opening and relaxing.
   * Finally, breathing steadily through your nose, concentrate on the sound of your own breathing for 5 minutes.

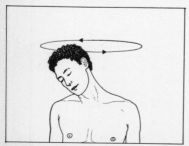

1) NECK ROLLS. Rotate the neck and head clockwise/anti-clockwise.

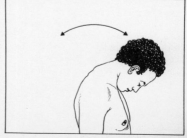

2) HEAD HANGS. Hang head forwards and hold, then backwards and hold.

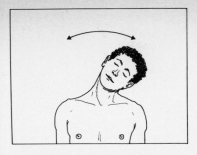

3) HEAD SWAYS. Tilt head to left and hold, then to right and hold.

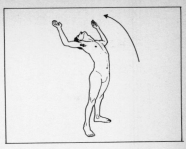

4) BACK ARCH. Arch body backwards so that it hangs, then hold.

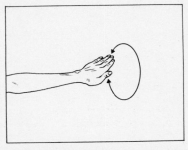

5) ARM ROTATION. Rotate left arm clockwise/anti-clockwise, then right arm.

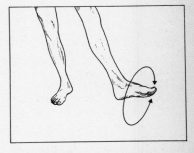

6) LEG ROTATION. Rotate left leg clockwise/anti-clockwise, then right leg.

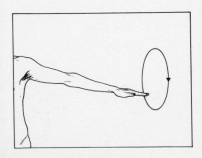

7) HAND ROTATION. Rotate left hand clockwise/anti-clockwise, then right hand.

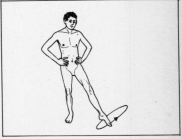

8) FOOT ROTATION. Rotate left foot clockwise/anti-clockwise, then right foot.

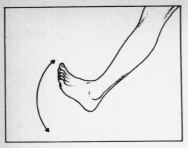

9) **TOE POINTS.** Point toes forwards and hold, then backwards and hold. Relax.

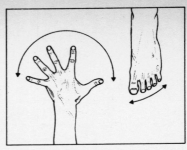

10) **FINGER & TOE STRETCHES.** Stretch fingers apart and hold, then relax. Repeat with toes.

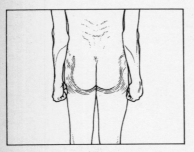

11) **FIST & BUTTOCK CLENCHES.** Clench fist and buttocks. Hold, then relax.

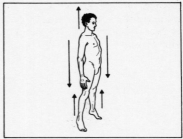

12) **BODY STRETCHES.** Force body upwards and shoulders and arms downwards. Relax.

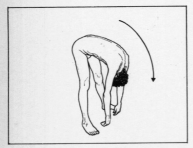

13) **BODY HANGS.** Bend forward to let upper body and arms hang loosely.

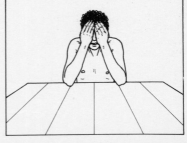

14) **EYE REST.** Rest head in hands and with palms cupped over eyes.

Qi Gong self-massage is a Chinese method of relaxing and refreshing the body to remedy stress and tiredness. It also improves circulation and stimulates internal organs. Qi Gong is quick and simple. It can be done almost anywhere – at home, during a tea break, or travelling on a train.

Instructions

1) Choose a quiet room.
2) Stand near an open window for fresh air.
3) Close your eyes.
4) Begin with 1 minute of deep breathing – inhaling and exhaling through your nose without holding your breath. Concentrate your mind on the sound and length of each breath.
5) Proceed to do the Qi Gong exercises – keeping your eyes closed as you do each one.

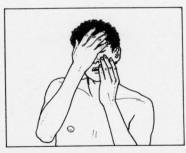

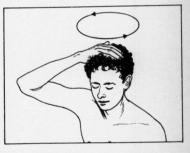

1) **DRY FACE WASH.** Rub the palms together briskly until they are hot. Then rub the face all over. Repeat 3x.

2) **SCALP MASSAGE.** Place the left palm on top of the head. With a circular movement, rub lightly clockwise. Then with the right palm, rub anti-clockwise. 10x each direction.

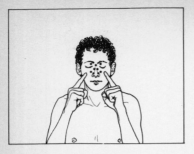

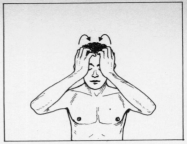

3) FINGER FACIAL. With the forefingers, in small circular motions firmly massage the nostrils, cheeks at the base of the nose, bridge of the nose, forehead between the eyes and the underside of the eyebrows.

4) SCALP BRUSHES. Bend the head forward. Press the fingertips firmly into the hairline and briefly hold. Then brush the fingers back through the hair to the nape of the neck. Repeat 5x.

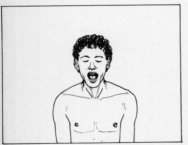

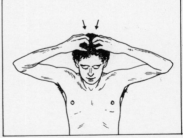

5) JAW STRETCHES. Stretch the jaws open as wide as possible and hold. Then relax. Click the teeth together 10x. Clench the teeth tightly together and hold. Then relax. Click the teeth together 10x. Repeat 3x.

6) SCALP PRESSES. Press the fingertips firmly into a line one inch on either side of the centre of the head and hold. Then beat along the line with the knuckles of both fists.

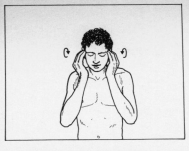
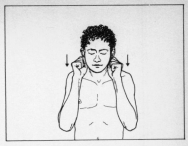

7) TEMPLE & FOREHEAD
MASSAGES. With the fingertips,
gently massage the temples in
small circular motions clockwise/
anti-clockwise 10x. Then massage
the forehead.

8) EAR PRESSURE & PULLS.
With the thumb and forefinger
squeeze the ears all over 20x. Then
pull both earlobes firmly
downwards 20x.

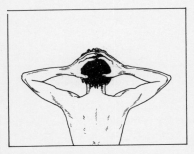
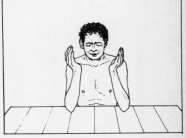

9) BACK OF THE HEAD
MASSAGE. Bend the head
forward. Massage the two bony
bumps at the back of the head.
Then press the fingertips firmly
and rhythmically along the vertical
neck muscles.

10) EYE REFRESHER. Squeeze
the eyes tightly shut and hold.
Relax. Repeat 5x. Then cup the
hands in front of the face. Bend
forward and gently rest the eyes in
the palms for 60 seconds.

Body massage is a great way of *sharing* relaxation with your lover or favourite friend. It can be used as a method for reducing tension and ensuring a relaxed sleep, or as an erotic prelude to sex.

Technique

1) To get clean and relaxed, take a hot shower or bath – together!
2) After drying off, spread a towel over the bed/floor to absorb any excess massage oil.
3) The person to be massaged should lie down, close their eyes, and do a minute of deep breathing to further relax.
4) The person massaging should then apply oil to the body (baby oil and some types of body lotions are suitable, or you can make your own using natural oils and herbal scents obtainable from a health food store).
5) Massage alternately using different parts of the hand – open palm, knuckles, heel of hand, finger and thumb tips and side of hand.
6) Vary massage methods between direct downwards pressure, circular motions, lengthways movements, rapid rhythmic on-off pressure, kneading and the pressing of flesh outwards from the centre of the body.
7) Intersperse massage with:
   – gentle caresses which barely touch the hairs on the body;
   – light pinches, scratches, bites and smacks.
8) For erotic effect, pay particular attention to the back of the neck, earlobes, nipples, waist, groin, buttocks, inside of arms and thighs, ankles, fingers, toes and soles of feet.
9) Conclude by briskly rubbing off oil with a towel. Then run the tongue over the body and breathe gently on the moistened areas.
10) Roll the body over and massage the other side.

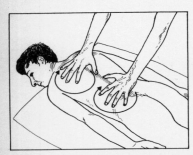

1) OPEN HAND. Circular movements with moderate pressure.

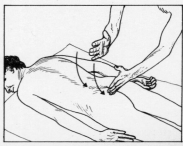

2) KARATE CHOPS. Rapid light chops lengthways along body.

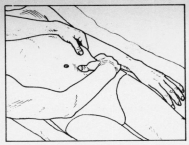

3) FINGER KNEADING. Finger manipulation as if kneading dough.

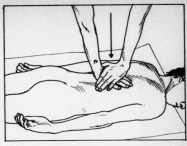

4) BODY WEIGHT PRESSURE. Along centre of back.

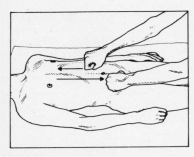

5) KNUCKLE RUBS. Using clenched fists.

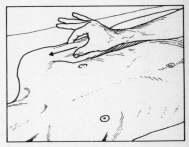

6) THUMB & FORE-FINGER GROOVING. Especially along arms and legs.

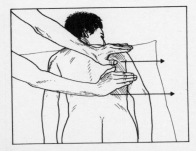

7) HEEL OF HAND. Press flesh outwards from the centre of body.

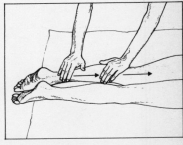

8) BRISK RUBBING. To create friction and heat.

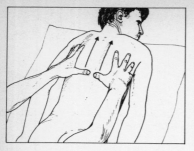

9) THUMB PAD PRESSURE.
Especially up and down spine.

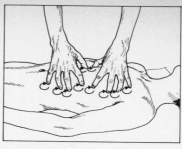

10) FINGERTIP ROTATIONS.
With fingers separated or bunched together.

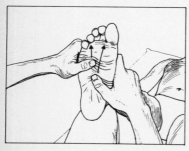

11) FEET. Strong thumb pressure on soles and between the toes.

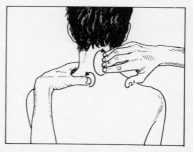

12) NECK & SHOULDERS.
Firm pressure in small rotating movements.

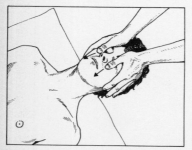

13) FACE. Press outwards from centre of face and delicately caress.

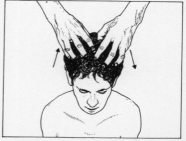

14) SCALP. Massage vigorously, scratch lightly and gently pull hair.

Appendix 9
Acupressure

Acupressure can help relieve tension, pain and minor ailments. Whenever there are two paired points on both sides of the body, always treat both simultaneously (except points on the hand which can obviously be treated only one at a time).

Technique

1) Locate appropriate acupressure points (usually indicated by soreness).
2) Apply pads of forefingers or thumbs (at points on earlobe and finger, squeeze between forefinger and tip of thumb).
3) Close eyes.
4) Use either (a) constant direct pressure, (b) rapid rhythmic on-off pressure, (c) massage pressure in small fast circular motions.
5) Begin with moderate pressure. Progress to strong pressure if needed.
6) Maintain pressure for 1–6 minutes.
7) Repeat as often as required.

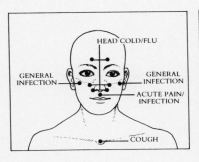

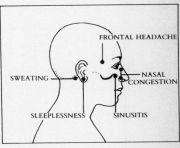

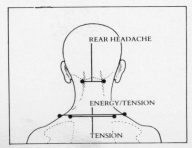

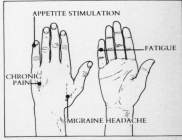

Useful contacts

The Terrence Higgins Trust

A registered charity to inform, advise and help on AIDS.
Helpline – (01) 833 2971 (7–10 pm weekdays & 3–10 pm weekends).

Body Positive

Body Positive is a self-help and mutual support group for people who are HTLV–3 antibody positive. For details of meetings, discos and other activities, phone Gay Switchboard or the Terrence Higgins Trust, who can also provide details of local AIDS helplines and counselling services.

Gay Switchboard

(01) 837 7324 (24 hours); BM Switchboard, London WC1N 3XX.

Haemophilia Society

(01) 407 1010; P.O. Box 9, 16 Trinity Street, London SE1 1DE.

I wish to make a donation to the fight against AIDS and help the work of the Terrence Higgins Trust.

Name .... Address ....

....

I enclose the donation of:
    £5 ☐   £10 ☐   £15 ☐   £20 ☐   £25 ☐   £50 ☐

Return to: The Terrence Higgins Trust, BM AIDS, London WC1N 3XX.